Viral Outbreaks: 2019-2023 Overview

Edited By

Amandeep Singh
Department of Pharmaceutics
ISF College of Pharmacy
Moga, Punjab, India

Viral Outbreaks: 2019-2023 Overview

Editor: Amandeep Singh

ISBN (Online): 978-981-5313-47-5

ISBN (Print): 978-981-5313-48-2

ISBN (Paperback): 978-981-5313-49-9

First published in 2025.

need for a court order if at any point you breach any terms of this License Agreement. In no event will any delay or failure by Bentham Science Publishers in enforcing your compliance with this License Agreement constitute a waiver of any of its rights.

3. You acknowledge that you have read this License Agreement, and agree to be bound by its terms and conditions. To the extent that any other terms and conditions presented on any website of Bentham Science Publishers conflict with, or are inconsistent with, the terms and conditions set out in this License Agreement, you acknowledge that the terms and conditions set out in this License Agreement shall prevail.

Bentham Science Publishers Pte. Ltd.
80 Robinson Road #02-00
Singapore 068898
Singapore
Email: subscriptions@benthamscience.net

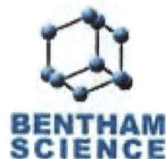

BENTHAM SCIENCE

CONTENTS

Navneet Arora, Rakesh Chawla, Abhishek Vijukumar, Amandeep Singh and *Ranjeet Kumar*

PREFACE 1

The past few years have been a period of unprecedented global health challenges, with viral outbreaks affecting every corner of the world. "Viral Outbreaks: 2019-2023 Overview" is a comprehensive account of these significant events, aiming to provide readers with a detailed understanding of the various viruses that have emerged and re-emerged during this time.

This book was conceived with the intention of documenting the characteristics, features, prevalence, number of cases, treatment options, and World Health Organization (WHO) recommendations for each major viral outbreak. The period from 2019 to 2023 has seen the world grapple with the devastating impacts of SARS-CoV-2 (COVID-19), as well as other significant viruses such as various strains of influenza, Dengue, Zika, H1N1 (Swine Flu), H5N8 (Avian Influenza), Ebola, and Lassa Fever. Each chapter provides a comprehensive overview of these outbreaks, presenting the latest data and insights into their management and control.

The COVID-19 pandemic, in particular, has highlighted the importance of global collaboration and the need for robust health infrastructures. The rapid spread of this novel coronavirus has had profound implications, not only for public health but also for economies, societies, and daily life. This book explores the multifaceted response to COVID-19, including the development of vaccines, therapeutic measures, and public health strategies, providing a detailed analysis of the global effort to combat this virus. In addition to COVID-19, the book delves into other viral threats that have posed significant challenges to public health. The chapters on influenza viruses, Dengue, Zika, H1N1, H5N8, Ebola, and Lassa Fever provide insights into the epidemiological characteristics, transmission dynamics, clinical features, and the global response to these viruses. By examining these diverse outbreaks, the book underscores the continuous and evolving nature of viral threats and the need for ongoing vigilance and preparedness.

A significant aspect of this book is its focus on WHO recommendations. The WHO has played a crucial role in guiding the global response to these outbreaks, providing essential guidelines, coordinating international efforts, and promoting research and development. This book highlights the WHO's contributions and the importance of adhering to their recommendations to mitigate the impact of viral outbreaks.

I would like to express my gratitude to all the researchers, and healthcare professionals, who have contributed to our understanding of these viruses and to the ongoing efforts to combat them. Their dedication and hard work have been instrumental in advancing our knowledge and improving our response to viral outbreaks.

As you read through this book, I hope you gain a deeper understanding of the complexities and challenges involved in managing viral outbreaks. It is my hope that this knowledge will inspire continued efforts to improve global health and prepare for future pandemics.

Amandeep Singh
Department of Pharmaceutics
ISF College of Pharmacy
Moga, Punjab, India

PREFACE 2

The period from 2019 to 2023 has been marked by a series of significant viral outbreaks, each posing unique challenges to global health systems and societies at large. This book, "Viral Outbreaks: 2019-2023 Overview," aims to provide a comprehensive account of these outbreaks, focusing on the characteristics, prevalence, treatment options, and the World Health Organization's (WHO) recommendations for each virus.

As we navigate through the intricacies of these outbreaks, it becomes evident that our world is increasingly interconnected, making the spread of infectious diseases a global concern rather than a localized issue. The COVID-19 pandemic, caused by the SARS-CoV-2 virus, is a stark reminder of how rapidly a virus can proliferate and disrupt lives, economies, and healthcare systems worldwide. This book delves into the multifaceted nature of COVID-19, exploring its unprecedented impact and the collaborative efforts undertaken to combat it.

In addition to COVID-19, this book also covers other significant viral threats, including various influenza viruses, Dengue, Zika, H1N1 (Swine Flu), H5N8 (Avian Influenza), Ebola, and Lassa Fever. Each chapter meticulously details the epidemiological characteristics, transmission methods, clinical features, and global response to these viruses. By presenting these diverse outbreaks in one volume, the book highlights the continuous and evolving challenge posed by viral diseases.

A key component of this book is the emphasis on WHO recommendations. The WHO has been at the forefront of global health, providing guidelines and coordinating international efforts to manage and mitigate the impact of viral outbreaks. Their role in shaping public health policies, spearheading vaccination campaigns, and promoting research and development is critically examined throughout the chapters.

The goal of this book is not only to document the events of the past few years but also to derive valuable lessons that can inform future responses to similar threats. It underscores the importance of preparedness, timely intervention, and international cooperation in combating viral outbreaks. The insights provided here aim to contribute to a better understanding of how we can improve our defences against future pandemics, ensuring a more resilient and responsive global health infrastructure.

As you delve into this comprehensive overview, we hope you gain a deeper appreciation of the complexities involved in managing viral outbreaks and the concerted efforts required to protect public health. This book serves as a testament to the resilience of humanity in the face of adversity and a call to action for continued vigilance and innovation in the field of infectious diseases.

Amandeep Singh
Department of Pharmaceutics
ISF College of Pharmacy
Moga, Punjab, India

List of Contributors

Ayushreeya Banga — Department of Pharmacy Practice, ISF College of Pharmacy, Moga, Punjab-142001, India

Anish Soni — Department of Pharmaceutical Analysis, ISF College of Pharmacy, Moga, Punjab-142001, India

Akshita Arora — Department of Pharmaceutics, ISF College of Pharmacy, Moga, Punjab-142001, India

Amandeep Singh — Department of Pharmaceutics, ISF College of Pharmacy, Moga, Punjab-142001, India

Ashmeen Kaur — Department of Pharmacy Practice, ISF College of Pharmacy, Moga, Punjab-142001, India

Animesh Ranjan — Department of Regulatory Affairs, ISF College of Pharmacy, Moga, Punjab-142001, India

Abhishek Vijukumar — Department of Pharmacy Practice, I.S.F College of Pharmacy, Moga, Punjab-142001, India

Bharat Sharma — Department of Pharmaceutical Analysis, ISF College of Pharmacy, Moga, Punjab-142001, India

Brajesh Kumar Panda — Department of Quality Assurance, ISF College of Pharmacy, Moga, Punjab-142001, India

Dilpreet Singh — University Institute of Pharma Sciences, Chandigarh University, Gharuan-140413, India

Deepak Singh Bisht — Department of Pharmaceutical Chemistry, ISF College of Pharmacy, Moga, Punjab-142001, India

Diksha — Department of Quality Assurance, ISF College of Pharmacy, Moga, Punjab-142001, India

Dhritisri Dutta — Department of Pharmacy Practice, ISF College of Pharmacy, Moga, Punjab-142001, India

Gurmeet Singh — Department of Pharmaceutics, ISF College of Pharmacy, Moga, Punjab-142001, India

Harshitha Mathur — Department of Pharmaceutics, ISF College of Pharmacy, Moga, Punjab-142001, India

Komal Mahajan — Department of Pharmaceutics, ISF College of Pharmacy, Moga, Punjab-142001, India

Naresh Kumar Rangra — Chitkara University School of Pharmacy, Chitkara University, Baddi, Himachal Pradesh, India

Nitin Sharma — Department of Pharmaceutics, Amity Institute of Pharmacy, Amity University, Noida-201301, India

Neeraj Patil — Department of Regulatory Affairs, ISF College of Pharmacy, Moga, Punjab-142001, India

Navneet Arora — Department of Pharmacy Practice, I.S.F College of Pharmacy, Moga, Punjab-142001, India

Prabhjot Kaur   Department of Pharmaceutical Chemistry, ISF College of Pharmacy, Moga, Punjab-142001, India

Prabhjot Kaur   Department of Food and Nutrition, Punjab Agricultural University, Ludhiana, Punjab-141004, India

Pawan Kumar   Department of Pharmaceutical Chemistry, ISF College of Pharmacy, Moga, Punjab-142001, India

Pooja Chawla   University Institute of Pharmaceutical Sciences and Research, Baba Farid University of Health Sciences, Faridkot, Punjab-151203, India

Rohit Bhatia   Department of Pharmaceutical Chemistry, ISF College of Pharmacy, Moga, Punjab-142001, India

Rojin G. Raj   Department of Pharmacy Practice, ISF College of Pharmacy, Moga, Punjab-142001, India

Rakesh Chawla   Department of Pharma Chemistry, University Institute of Pharmacy, Baba Farid University of Health Sciences, Faridkot, Punjab-151203, India

Ranjeet Kumar   Department of Pharmacy Practice, I.S.F College of Pharmacy, Moga, Punjab-142001, India

Shalini Jaswal   Department of Pharmaceutical Chemistry, ISF College of Pharmacy, Moga, Punjab-142001, India

Subramanya Sarma Ganti   Department of Pharmaceutical Chemistry, ISF College of Pharmacy, Moga, Punjab-142001, India

Simranjeet Kaur   Department of Pharmaceutics, ISF College of Pharmacy, Moga, Punjab-142001, India

Tuhin James Paul   Department of Pharmacy Practice, ISF College of Pharmacy, Moga, Punjab-142001, India

CHAPTER 1

The Outbreak of Various Viral Diseases from 2019-2023

Harshitha Mathur[1], Shalini Jaswal[2], Tuhin James Paul[3], Ayushreeya Banga[3], Subrahmanya Sarma Ganti[2] and Rohit Bhatia[2,*]

[1] *Department of Pharmaceutics, ISF College of Pharmacy, Moga, Punjab-142001, India*

[2] *Department of Pharmaceutical Chemistry, ISF College of Pharmacy, Moga, Punjab-142001, India*

[3] *Department of Pharmacy Practice, ISF College of Pharmacy, Moga, Punjab-142001, India*

Abstract: In this chapter, recent viral disease outbreaks—especially those that happened in 2019 and 2023—are thoroughly examined. The chapter also highlights the burden that both emerging and re-emerging viral threats place on healthcare systems globally, as well as the challenges that these threats pose to human and animal health globally. The analysis explores mechanisms such as genetic reassortment, increased human-animal interaction, and the impact of globalization that contribute to the emergence and spread of viruses. The transmission dynamics, clinical manifestations, and diagnostic difficulties related to a range of viral diseases—including respiratory infections as well as those affecting the liver, circulatory system, spleen, and pancreas—are also discussed in the article. Research is also conducted on the immune system's function in preventing viral infections, specifically on the roles of innate and adaptive immunity. Moreover, the significance of strong surveillance frameworks, efficient infection control protocols, and non-pharmaceutical strategies such as physical distancing and travel limitations in managing viral epidemics is underscored. The chapter recognizes the difficulties that pandemics present for healthcare systems, emphasizing the necessity of sufficient equipment, personnel, and clinical management techniques. It also highlights the need for emergency preparedness plans in order to lessen the wider economic and social effects of viral outbreaks and investigates the potential of telemedicine as a useful tool.

Keywords: Emerging infectious diseases, Re-emerging viruses, Respiratory viral infections, Viral outbreaks.

---

* **Corresponding author Rohit Bhatia:** Department of Pharmaceutical Chemistry, ISF College of Pharmacy, Moga, Punjab-142001, India; E-mail: bhatiarohit5678@gmail.com

Amandeep Singh (Ed.)

INTRODUCTION

Throughout history, viral outbreaks have been a recurrent phenomenon, albeit with varying degrees of severity. Genetic reassortment events frequently give rise to novel viral strains, which can lead to outbreaks with epidemic or epidemic eventuality. Humanity frequently finds itself ill-set to combat these imperative pitfalls. The early 21st century is known for several notable afflictions, which include severe acute respiratory pattern coronavirus (SARS- CoV), Middle East respiratory pattern coronavirus (MERS- CoV), and SARS- CoV- 2, along with new influenzas similar as avian and swine flu. These outbreaks have originated from specific geographical regions but have swiftly spread across the globe, wreaking havoc across all sectors. Infectious diseases continue to stand as primary contributors to human and animal morbidity and mortality, resulting in substantial healthcare expenditures globally. The world has witnessed numerous outbreaks and epidemics of various infectious diseases, underscoring the ongoing challenge they pose to public health and healthcare systems worldwide [1]. The diverse geographical and climatic conditions, coupled with uneven population distribution, create distinct patterns in the spread of viral diseases within the country. Various biological, socio-cultural, and ecological factors, alongside new dynamics in human-animal interactions, further complicate the emergence of infectious diseases. Addressing these challenges in controlling and preventing both emerging and recurring infectious diseases requires a comprehensive understanding of the underlying factors contributing to their emergence, as well as the establishment of robust surveillance systems aimed at reducing human casualties and fatalities [2]. The trajectory of new infections typically unfolds in a sequence, starting with their emergence, then transitioning into local transmission, expanding across borders, and potentially culminating in global spread. Various global shifts can influence the likelihood of emergence, the dynamics of disease within local communities, and the extent to which diseases spread between different populations [3]. The ubiquity of phrases like "going viral" often obscures the precise scientific meaning of viruses, a fact sometimes overlooked by the general public. In everyday language, viruses are often conflated with any unseen germ, much to the chagrin of virologists. While this lack of specificity may not seem consequential, it becomes problematic when it leads to the misuse of antibiotics, which are ineffective against viruses but target bacteria instead [4]. Frequently depicted as entities teetering on the edge of life, viruses exist in various relationships with living organisms, ranging from parasitic to commensal or even symbiotic. They are present across the spectrum of life forms, from single-celled Archaea and bacteria to plants, animals, and humans. Viruses serve a dual purpose in laboratory settings, serving as subjects of study and as tools for experimentation. They have significantly deepened our comprehension, not just of human illnesses, but also of the broader living ecosystem [4]. Patients can acquire viral infections through direct exposure to infected materials or through viral reactivation. In transplant units, where the risk of transmission is high, it is crucial for facilities to establish and follow documented infection control procedures. These protocols should include measures such as thorough hand washing, regular cleaning of medical equipment like stethoscopes, adherence to droplet precautions, and effective patient isolation techniques. By universally adhering to these guidelines, the spread of nosocomial infections can be significantly reduced [5]. Over the past decade, there have been several significant global outbreaks of infectious diseases that posed substantial health risks. Numerous of these fleetly spreading contagions, similar to avian influenza and SARS, seem to have started as zoonotic conditions in Asia [6]. The constant trouble of morbidity and mortality from arising contagious conditions is conceded, although the precise extent of this trouble remains unclear. A widely recognized definition, proposed by the Institute of Medicine (IOM) in the United States in 1992, describes an emerging contagious disease as a new, reemerging, or medication-resistant infection whose prevalence in humans has increased over the past 20 years or is expected to rise in the near future [7]. There exists a diapason of pathogens that crop and spread among populations. This broad spectrum includes animal-borne infectious diseases such as SARS, which have recently been linked to human illness, and genetically modified organisms that create conditions in unexpected ways, such as the 2001 anthrax outbreak in the United States that was spread through contaminated correspondence. Indeed, failures in fundamental measures for public health, such as the treatment of existing infections (*e.g.*, tuberculosis) or routine non-age immunisations (*e.g.*, poliomyelitis), may cause a resurgence of conditions that were previously thought to be under control. Additionally, this chain of events includes the appearance of newer disease strains that are resistant to antibiotics yet continue to pose a threat, like the methicillin-resistant *Staphylococcus aureus* [8]. The 21st century is characterized by significant pandemics, including epidemics, caused by both traditional conditions like pests, cholera, and yellow fever, as well as the rising ones analogous to a severe acute respiratory cycle (SARS), Zika, Ebola, Middle East respiratory pattern (MERS), HIV (although technically endemic), influenza A(H1N1) p.m./ 09, and utmost recently, COVID- 19. Multifold of these contagions primarily affects the respiratory system. Despite developments in drugs, tuberculosis (TB), which killed 1.5 million people in 2018, continues to be the most common infectious complaint attributed to a single organism [9].

The influenza virus has a major impact on the lungs because it can cause pneumonia and aggravate already existing lung diseases [10]. Occurrences of such events are typically infrequent and fluctuate throughout most seasonal influenza periods, yet they can become more prevalent and intense during pandemics. For instance, in the 2018–2019 season, in the USA, approximately 32 million influenza cases were reported, leading to an estimated 32,000 deaths [11]. The H1N1 virus, responsible for the pandemics of 1918 and 2009, demonstrates a tendency to induce swifter and more severe pneumonia compared to other strains, often leading to elevated instances of bacterial superinfection [12].

Viral Diseases of the Lung

Respiratory infections caused by viruses pose significant public health challenges as they can easily spread from one person to another through various means. These include direct transmission *via* aerosols, small Driblets, or contagion-laden secretions, as well as circular transmission through contact with defiled shells [13]. Respiratory driblets, particularly those of significant size, are predominantly produced during activities such as coughing, sneezing, and talking, as well as medical procedures like suctioning and bronchoscopy, which can also generate smaller droplets known as droplet nuclei. These microorganisms become airborne when expelled by an infected individual and can be deposited on others' conjunctivae, nasal mucosa, or mouth, leading to transmission. Larger droplets tend to fall rapidly onto nearby surfaces, heightening the risk of transmission through contact. Additionally, viral infections can spread through smaller aerosol particles, measuring less than 5-10 μm in size, which may remain infectious over longer distances, extending up to several meters [14]. Emerging evidence indicates that the SARS coronavirus 2 (SARS-CoV-2) virus could potentially be detected in exhaled air during routine activities such as talking and breathing [15] and has been found to persist on various surfaces for several hours [16]. Respiratory infections can be distributed clinically depending on the pattern observed or based on the virus causing them (much like influenza). Symptoms typically include fever, sneezing, runny nose, dry cough, breathing difficulties, muscle aches, exhaustion, and throat inflammation without pus formation [17]. The clinical spectrum might encompass cases with no symptoms, infections of the upper and lower respiratory tracts that can lead to pneumonia, acute respiratory distress syndrome, and complete body infection [18]. Viral respiratory diseases can vary widely in severity, and older people are more likely to develop a severe illness regardless of other medical issues. Infants, on the other hand, may suffer more severely from certain pathogens. Morbidity can stem directly from viral infection or arise from the worsening of pre-existing medical conditions or secondary bacterial infections [19, 20]. Variations in population demographics, geographic features, climate conditions, vaccination rates, and socioeconomic position lead to differences in the transmission patterns of respiratory virus infections between nations and regions [21].

Viral Diseases of other Organs

Our bodies are like intricate ecosystems, where every organ works together seamlessly to keep us healthy. While we often associate viruses with respiratory illnesses like the common cold or influenza, these microscopic invaders can pose a significant threat to various internal organs as well [22, 23]. From the liver, responsible for detoxification and metabolism, to the spleen, a vital part of the immune system, no organ is immune to viral attacks. The pancreas, crucial for digestion and blood sugar regulation, and the intricate network of the circulatory system can also be compromised by viral infections. Understanding these potential threats and the specific viruses that target these organs is essential for promoting preventive measures and early intervention [24].

Viral Diseases of the Liver

While viral hepatitis often takes center stage when discussing viruses and the liver, a lesser-known threat also emerges during Dengue illness outbreaks. This section highlights liver involvement in adults with Dengue Illness (DI) and Viral Hepatitis Infection [25]. The key takeaway is that liver injury is extremely common in adult DI and Viral Hepatitis patients. This differs from children with DI, where liver problems tend to be more frequent and severe. Interestingly, liver injury in adults with DI mimicked viral hepatitis [26]. However, specific tests can help distinguish between the two conditions such as the presence of thrombocytopenia and persistent fever even after jaundice signify DI. Serological tests such as blood tests that detect specific antibodies or viral components, can further solidify the diagnosis. The tests would look for antibodies against hepatotropic viruses, while another test would specifically check for Dengue virus thus confirming the disease. Another potential complication - ascites, a buildup of fluid in the abdomen is observed in DI patients and might be linked to increased pressure in a vein connected to the liver [27]. Rudbar *et al.*, explained the clinical symptoms of dengue illness as pleural effusion, ascites, hemorrhage, breathlessness, bleeding gums, hepatomegaly, and splenomegaly [28]. Every year, viral hepatitis tragically takes the lives of 1.34 million people worldwide. Hepatitis B infection is the leading cause, accounting for over 884,000 deaths. Hepatitis C is another major threat, causing 400,000 deaths annually. Hepatitis E contributes to 69,000 deaths, and Hepatitis A, though less deadly, claims around 32,245 lives each year. Clearly, the major portion of the deaths (about 96%) are caused by HBV and HCV infections, therefore major health surveillance and screening programs focus on tackling HBV and HCV infection [29]. Clinical symptoms for viral hepatitis are like the dengue illness but differ in showing symptoms of Thrombocytopenia and fever after jaundice. Currently, two main medication types are approved for treating chronic Hepatitis B (HBV) and

Hepatitis C (HCV) infection: interferon-alpha (IFN) drugs and nucleoside/nucleotide analogues (NAs) [30]. These drugs have brought down the mortality rate for acute hepatitis infection but still, a substantial decline in mortality is yet to be seen [31]. Fig. (1), explains the Immuno-Vascular nature of Dengue Virus (DENV) infection [32].

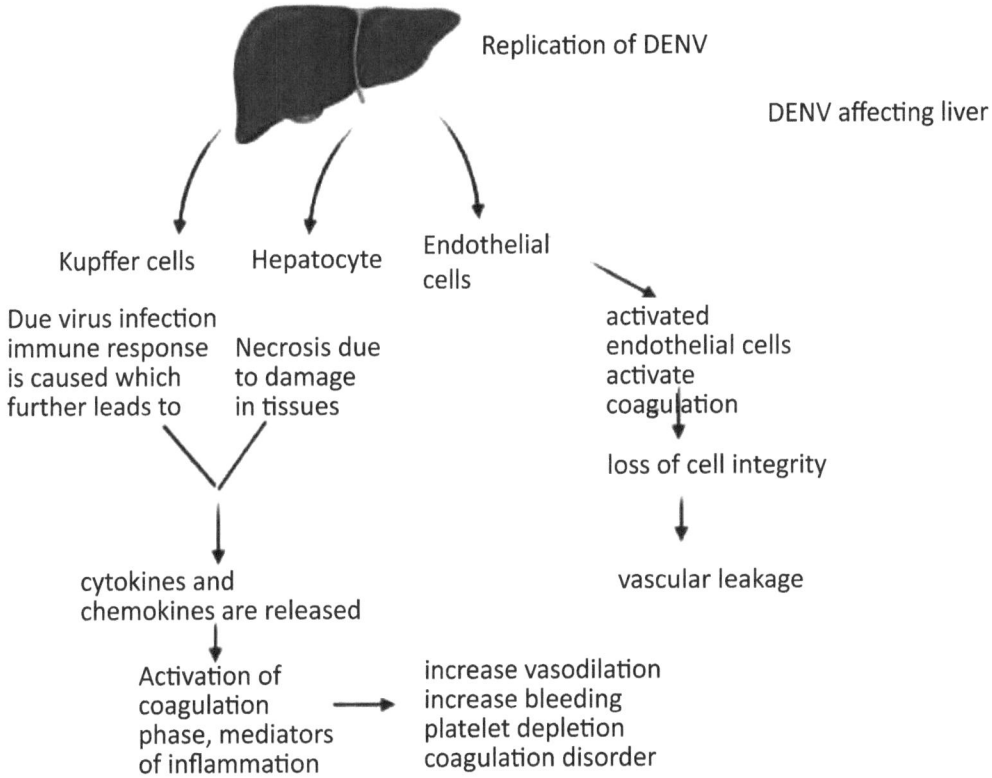

Fig. (1). DENV affecting liver [32].

Viral Diseases of the Circulatory System

Blood transfusions are a cornerstone of modern medicine, but they can also carry the hidden threat of transmitting infectious agents. In recent years, the emergence of arboviruses – mosquito-vector viruses like chikungunya (CHIKV), dengue (DENV), and Zika (ZIKV) – has heightened concerns about blood safety. A major challenge lies in the potential for asymptomatic, infected donors to unwittingly transmit these viruses. Studies employing highly sensitive NAT (nucleic acid testing) revealed alarmingly high viremic rates (presence of virus particles) in outbreak areas – up to 5.5% for DENV [32 - 34]. These infected individuals pose a significant risk as they may not exhibit any symptoms of the disease. Unfortunately, NAT testing remains expensive and not universally available.

Most countries lack the resources to routinely implement it for blood donor screening. Another approach relies on assessing seroprevalence, the presence of antibodies indicating past exposure to a virus [35]. Studies have shown high seroprevalence rates for CHIKV and DENV, particularly in areas with frequent outbreaks. However, seroprevalence does not necessarily translate to current infection and risk of transmission. Several strategies can be implemented to minimize the risk of arbovirus transmission through blood transfusions. (A) Asking blood donors targeted questions about recent symptoms and encouraging them to report any health concerns after donation can help identify potential infections, (B) Delaying the release of red blood cell concentrates until after the incubation period for arboviruses has passed could offer an additional layer of protection, (C) Implementing rapid and affordable tests for CHIKV, DENV, and ZIKV at blood donation centers could be a valuable tool. These methods have proven effective against various arboviruses and could offer an additional level of safety. The success of these approaches hinges on several factors. One is how readily available resources are, such as funding and testing equipment. Another is the accuracy of the tests themselves. Finally, it is important to consider whether the tests can accurately distinguish between different arboviruses, as they may have similar characteristics. Additionally, studies reviewed here may not be fully illustrative of the general population due to geographical and prevalence differences [36]. The emergence of COVID-19 has presented unique challenges, particularly for elderly patients. This provides two concerning trends that may worsen outcomes in this vulnerable population. Our bodies possess a natural defense mechanism called neutrophilic extracellular trap (NET) formation or Enosis. While this process helps eliminate pathogens, excessive NET formation can damage surrounding tissues. Research suggests a potential link between excessive Enosis and the development of severe COVID-19 complications, such as lung, heart, and kidney problems, in elderly patients. Further investigation into NET formation within the context of COVID-19 is necessary. Additionally, therapies that target NETs hold promise in mitigating the damage caused by the body's overreaction to the virus [37]. Elderly COVID-19 patients, especially those presenting with neurological symptoms, may be more susceptible to hemorrhagic stroke, a type of stroke caused by bleeding in the brain. The exact mechanism behind this increased risk is still unclear, but it might involve changes in hormone levels triggered by the virus binding to specific receptors. These changes could lead to high blood pressure, increased blood vessel permeability, and impaired blood vessel function – all factors contributing to hemorrhagic stroke. Underlying hypertension is a significant risk factor, and COVID-19 patients with high blood pressure are particularly vulnerable. Furthermore, the overactive immune response often seen in COVID-19, coupled with stress and anxiety in these patients, could further increase stroke risk by affecting blood flow in the brain [38, 39].

Viral Diseases of the Spleen

The impact of **severe acute respiratory syndrome** (SARS) on the spleen, a vital organ in the immune system remains profound [40]. Researchers examined spleen tissue from deceased SARS patients and revealed significant damage to immune cells. The evidence suggests a direct attack by the SARS virus, infecting and harming various immune cell types within the spleen. These include lymphocytes (T cells and B cells) and dendritic cells. The presence of the virus in these cells and the drop in their figures compared to healthy individualities support this notion. The widespread destruction of immune cells in the spleen likely contributes to the weakened immune system observed in SARS patients [41]. This may explain why some patients develop opportunistic infections later in the course of the disease. While the exact way the SARS virus damages immune cells remains unclear, researchers suspect a common mechanism for different cell types. This mechanism may involve dendritic cells causing the infection to be an immune-deficient and immune-over-reaction. Notably, steroid treatment was not responsible for the decline in immune cell numbers, which is sometimes used to manage SARS symptoms. The severity of immune system damage appeared to be linked to the duration of the illness. Patients who battled the disease for longer periods exhibited a greater reduction in immune cell numbers. These findings suggest that SARS causes significant immune system injury, particularly in the spleen [42]. This damage likely plays a crucial part in the complaint's progression and may explain the characteristic lymphopenia observed in SARS cases. Understanding how the virus harms the immune system could be crucial for developing better treatments and understanding SARS pathogenesis [43, 44].

Viral Diseases of the Pancreas

Acute pancreatitis (AP), a sudden inflammation of the pancreas, is most commonly caused by alcohol or gallstones. However, viral infections can also play a role, and this area remains less understood. Simons Laures *et al.* aimed to shed light on the connection between viruses and AP [45]. Their analysis revealed some key points. First, there's a lack of comprehensive data on virus-induced AP using standardized diagnostic criteria. This makes it difficult to get a clear picture of the phenomenon. Second, a significant portion (28%) of patients with viral AP are immunocompromised. This number jumps to a staggering 71.4% among those who died. This suggests that a weakened immune system may be a critical factor influencing outcomes in viral AP [46]. Their study also found a higher mortality rate (20%) compared to what's typically reported for other causes of AP (5%). Exactly how viruses cause AP remains unclear. Some viruses may directly infect pancreatic cells, while others might trigger inflammation through mechanisms like blocked bile ducts [47]. The effectiveness of antiviral medications in treating viral AP is also uncertain. Decisions on antiviral therapy should be based on factors like the presence of disseminated viral infection and the patient's immune status. Diagnosing viral infections in older studies, before widespread PCR testing, might be less accurate. Additionally, many cases do not definitively exclude common causes of AP like alcohol or gallstones. Moving forward, larger studies with more patients are needed to get a better understanding of viral AP. Prospective studies that follow patients over time would provide valuable insights. Furthermore, research is needed to elucidate the mechanisms by which different viruses damage the pancreas. By addressing these knowledge gaps, researchers can improve diagnosis, treatment, and ultimately, outcomes for patients with viral AP [48]. The recent Outbreak of SARS COV2 greatly affected the Cardiovascular system (Lungs) and the Pancreas (Beta cells), Fig. (**2**) describes the pathogenesis descriptively [49].

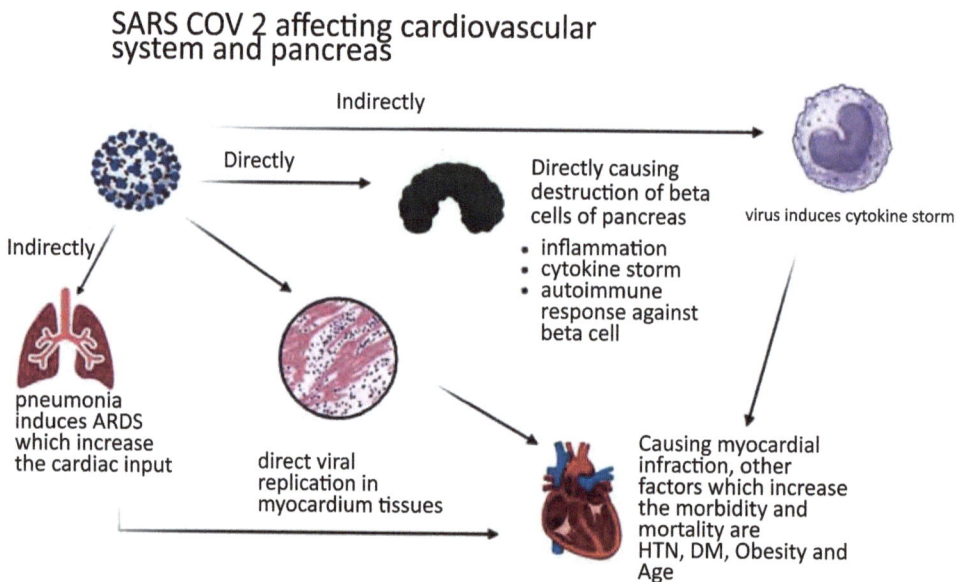

Fig. (2). SARS COV-2 affecting the cardiovascular system and pancreas [49].

Immunology

Our bodies have natural ways to fight off respiratory viruses, like mucus that traps them and special molecules that can inactivate them. But if these defenses aren't enough, viruses can infect cells by latching onto specific docking points (receptors) on the outside of those cells [50]. Ingrain vulnerable cells including dendritic cells, alveolar macrophages, natural killer cells, and neutrophils are mobilized in response to viral infections. These cells play crucial roles in initiating antiviral responses and facilitating the development of adaptive immunity. However, the inflammatory activity of these cells can also contribute to innate immune-mediated tissue damage, a phenomenon observed not only in viral infections but also in conditions like tuberculosis [51]. T- cells play a pivotal part in stimulating the B-cell response and cell- intermediated immunity, eventually assisting in the concurrence of contagions. Specifically, B-cells induce antibodies that can directly neutralize respiratory contagions by either binding to viral shell proteins or initiating the complement waterfall [52]. T-follicular coadjutor cells, a distinct subset of CD4 T- cells, are integral to the establishment of protective immunity by assisting B-cells in the production of antibodies against invading pathogens [53]. Viral elimination is facilitated by CD8+ T-cells possessing cytolytic capabilities. The immune response against viruses is predominantly driven by the T-helper cell type 1 (Th1) response, primarily *via* the production of interferon (IFN)-γ, which contributes to protective antiviral activity [54, 55]. Also, to alleviate cellular damage to lungs, these responses are precisely regulated. T-cells employ regulatory mechanisms similar to cytokine secretion and the increase of inhibitory receptors to finely modulate the vulnerable response [56], results in an increase of the T-regulatory cell subset plays a pivotal part in achieving a balance between tissue damage and viral concurrence. Likewise, the vulnerable systems of neonates, infants, children, and grown-ups display differences in both composition and functional responsiveness to contagious conditions [57, 58]. In the environment of Mycobacterium tuberculosis response, following the dispersion of mycobacteria up to the lymph node, dendritic cells expose bacterial antigens to T-cells and initiate their priming [59, 60]. Around 10 days post-infection, priming takes place in the mediastinal lymph bumps, eventually the generation of effector T-cells [61], and Th1 CD4 T-cells play a vital part in orchestrating the conformation of granulomas. Granulomas are organized structures wherein T-cells and B-cells enclose naturally vulnerable cells (macrophages and neutrophils) within a fibrotic capsule, creating a hypoxic atmosphere to stymie the growth of. Tuberculosis [62], still, hypoxia may complicate tissue destruction in tuberculosis [63]. In mouse studies, the part of CD8 T- cells in delivering safety against tuberculosis has been set up to be minor [64], likewise, there is an indeed lower contribution observed from B- cells and humoral impunity in providing protection against tuberculosis infection [65]. In discrepancy, mortal studies have linked tuberculosis-specific CD8 T-cells with active tuberculosis [66, 67], and this association has been observed in both HIV-uninfected and HIV-infected cases [68]. An elevated CD8 T-cell response has been identified with tuberculosis cargo and longitudinal studies have demonstrated a decline in this CD8 T-cell response during TB treatment [66].

Diagnostic Challenges in Viral Disease

There are many viruses responsible for severe acute respiratory infections [69] including SARS- CoV, MERS- CoV, and SARS- CoV- 2 [70 - 72]. To separate these viruses from similar bacterial infections, a planned lab methodology is essential. This strategy involves merging conventional virology assays with molecular levels that combine nucleic acid birth and PCR or RT PCR, along with the use of rapid molecular tests (RDTs) deployed in point-of-care minilabs. Favored results obtained through single or multiplex RDTs can facilitate appropriate cohosting and handling of infected patients [73]. Unfavored results are frequently inconclusive due to issues such as limited sensitivity and non-standardized specimen collection. Metagenomic next-generation sequencing can be utilized to detect pathogens not covered by conventional tests, including all viruses. Genomic data offers insights into virulence genes [74], and phylogenetic approaches are employed to identify resistance mutations and clusters within pathogen populations [75, 76]. The detection of specific antibodies continues to be valuable for conducting serum-prevalence studies in targeted populations and in vaccine research. The resurgence of previously known pathogens and the emergence of novel ones, such as SARS-CoV-2, underscore the critical significance of the global virus-checking program [77]. Table **1** provides list of all the diagnostic test available for each Viral Disease [73-77].

Table 1. List of all the diagnostic tests available for each viral disease.

Virus Name	Diagnostic Test
SARS-CoV	- RT-PCR (Reverse Transcription Polymerase Chain Reaction) - Antibody tests (ELISA, immunofluorescence assay ---- Viral culture
MERS-CoV	- RT-PCR -Serological tests (ELISA, immunofluorescence assay) - Virus isolation
SARS-CoV-2 (COVID-19)	- RT-PCR - Rapid antigen tests -Antibody tests (ELISA, lateral flow immunoassay)
Influenza viruses (including avian and swine flu	Rapid influenza diagnostic tests (RIDTs) - RT-PCR - Viral culture - Immunofluorescence assays
Zika virus	- RT-PCR - Serological tests (IgM ELISA, plaque reduction neutralization test)
Ebola virus	- RT-PCR -Antigen detection tests -Antibody tests (ELISA)

(Table 1) cont.....

Virus Name	Diagnostic Test
Yellow fever virus	- RT-PCR -Serological tests (IgM ELISA, plaque reduction neutralization test) -Virus isolation

CONTROLLING VIRAL DISEASE: STRENGTH AND OPPORTUNITIES

Principles of Viral Containment

Our interconnected world, with crowded cities and fast travel, allows viruses to spread quickly across continents in just hours. Since the 1918 flu pandemic, the main ways to fight new viruses haven't changed much. They focus on reducing exposure early on, like teaching good hygiene practices (coughing into elbows, washing hands) and encouraging people to stay home if sick. This can involve voluntary isolation of infected individuals or households, and quarantining their contacts. Later measures might include social distancing, travel restrictions, and public education campaigns. National lockdowns are a more extreme option to try and curb diseases like COVID-19, but they can wreck a country's economy. These non-drug interventions aim to slow the spread by reducing contact between people, bringing the virus's reproduction rate (R0) below 1. By lowering the number of sick people at the peak of the outbreak (flattening the curve), these measures ease the burden on hospitals and other essential services. While they may not stop everyone from getting sick, they buy time for developing and distributing vaccines and antiviral drugs. This approach also allows hospitals to prepare, acquire equipment, and develop better diagnostic tests.

Infection control is a crucial set of tactics to fight the spread of infections. It works in two main ways. Containment focuses on quickly identifying cases, isolating them to prevent further spread within the community, and tracking their contacts to monitor the situation. Imagine it like putting a lid on a pot to keep the infection from boiling over. Geographical restriction, on the other hand, aims to stop the infection from reaching new areas. This might involve creating a designated zone around an outbreak ("containment zone" or "cordon sanitaire") with stricter measures like increased testing and travel limitations. Additionally, they might monitor nearby areas ("buffer zone") to catch any cases that might spread beyond the initial zone [78, 79].

The key to slowing down an infection's spread is to find and treat cases early, track and check in with people who've been exposed, and keep people apart. This means limiting large gatherings, closing schools and businesses, and generally encouraging people to avoid contact. These measures aim to flatten the curve – reducing the number of sick people at any one time and keeping it within the capacity of hospitals. History backs this up. Cities that acted early during the 1918 flu pandemic saw far fewer deaths and less strain on their healthcare systems [80].

Airborne Infection Control and Workplace Safety

In healthcare settings, airborne infection control employs a scale of measures aimed at minimizing the threat of infection. This scale includes barring causes of infection, administering engineering controls, establishing administrative controls, and delivering protective outfits (*e.g.*, surgical masks for contagious cases and respirators for the healthcare labor force and guests) [81, 82]. For healthcare workers and others potentially exposed to hazardous airborne particles, wearing high-quality masks (like N95s) and eye protection is recommended after proper training. These masks offer much better protection than surgical masks, whose effectiveness is still being debated. While there's agreement regarding the use of surgical masks to limit the dissipation of drop centrals from insulated characteristic cases, the wide relinquishment of surgical masks to alleviate the community transmission of COVID-19, particularly during the early stages of infection and by asymptomatic individuals, is subject to intense debate [83, 84]. Opponents of widespread surgical mask use raise concerns about the false sense of security it may impart, where individuals mistakenly believe the mask offers complete protection against infection. Additionally, there are potential risks associated with moisture retention, extended mask reuse, and the limited filtration capacity of surgical masks [85]. As the World Health Organization (WHO) revises its recommendations, the application of masks among community members is witnessing evaluation [86]. According to recent guidance from the European Centre for Disease Prevention and Control (ECDC), face masks worn by the general population could potentially drop the transmission of infection within the community by reducing the release of respiratory driblets from infected individuals who are either symptomatic or asymptomatic [87]. The rearmost evidence explosively supports direct contact and respiratory driblets as the primary routes of transmission for SARS-CoV- 2 [88], also, underscores the significance of thorough environmental face cleaning using sanitarium-grade detergents and meticulous hand hygiene. Common disinfection procedures, similar to a 5- nanosecond contact with household bleach, effectively inactivate SARS- CoV- 2 [89]. The contagion can be effectively excluded by the following detergents ice-cold acetone (90 seconds), ice-cold acetone/ methanol admixture (40/60, 10 minutes), 70 ethanol (10 minutes), 100 ethanol (5 minutes), paraformaldehyde (2 minutes), and glutaraldehyde (2 minutes). Also, generally used brands of hand detergents also kill SARS-CoV within 30 seconds [90]. The guidance from the European Centre for Disease Prevention and Control (ECDC) regarding disinfection of surroundings in both healthcare and-nonhealthcare settings potentially defiled with SARS- CoV- 2 suggests using products with virucidal exertion that are certified in public requests. Alternately, a result of 0.05 sodium hypochlorite (diluted 1/100 from household bleach, typically starting at a concentration of 5%) is recommended. For surfaces susceptible to damage from sodium hypochlorite, products containing ethanol with a concentration of at least 70% can be utilized [91].

The virus can survive for up to 4 days outside the body, especially in loose stools that are not acidic [91]. It can last outside the body for a long time, over a week in mucus (like coughs or sneezes) and at least 4 days in urine, stool, and even blood, all at regular room temperature [89]. The virus can remain viable for up to 9 days in suspension, 60 hours in soil or water, and more than 1 day on hard surfaces like glass and metal [90], and can survive for up to 48 hours on plastic surfaces [92]. Human coronavirus 229E can retain its infectiousness on high-touch environmental surfaces such as polyvinylchloride, laminate, wood, and stainless steel for a minimum of 7 days under ambient temperature (24°C) and relative humidity conditions (around 50%) [93]. COVID-19 exhibits specific characteristics, including rapid spread with a short incubation period, resulting in exponential infection rates that affect thousands of individuals across all age groups [94].

Human Resources, Equipment, and New Approaches to Clinical Management

Primarily, the COVID-19 pandemic represents a health extremity [95]. Still, it is fleetly evolving into a profitable extremity as well. In a vicious cycle, the drop in profitable conditioning leads to reduced plutocrat rotation, duty earnings, and budgeting available for enforcement of the essential public health measures to limit the epidemic. Government programs to help workers during economic downturns strain budgets. This poverty caused by the downturn will likely have negative effects on people's health, especially in poor countries. These effects include malnutrition and more diseases like TB. To address these current and future problems, countries need well-funded plans [96]. By making telehealth routine, we can avoid taking away resources from existing programs (like TB) to fight emergencies (like COVID-19). This includes things like PCR test kits, which are used for both diseases. A good emergency plan should make sure we can quickly get the tests, medicine, breathing machines, masks, protective gear, and staff we need to respond effectively [97, 98]. Table **2** provides the list of vaccines available for prevention of Viral disease for both Humans and animals [95-98].

Table 2. Vaccines available for prevention of viral disease in both humans and animals.

Virus Name	Human Vaccines	Animal Vaccines
COVID-19	Comirnaty (Pfizer-BioNTech), Spikevax (Moderna), Vaxzevria (AstraZeneca), Janssen COVID-19 Vaccine	Zoetis COVID-19 vaccine
Influenza	Fluzone, Fluarix, FluLaval, Flucelvax, FluMist	Fluvac Innovator, Prestige, Calvenza (for horses), Nobivac Canine Flu (for dogs)
Avian Influenza	No widespread human vaccine	Poulvac Flufend AI H5N3 RG, Nobilis Influenza H5N2
Zika virus	No approved vaccine	No approved vaccine

Telemedicine emerges as a vital approach for delivering care, particularly to mitigate the risk of infection associated with in-person contact [99]. For telehealth to be truly useful in emergencies, it needs to become a normal part of how healthcare works every day. This means revamping how things are run and changing the current ways we deliver care [100]. Table **3** describes the surveillance and other strategies adopted to manage the outbreaks in Humans and animals [99-100].

Table 3. Surveillance and other strategies adopted for managing the outbreak in humans and animals.

Strategy	Description
Surveillance Systems	Establish robust surveillance systems aimed at reducing human casualties and fatalities.
Comprehensive Understanding	Develop a thorough understanding of factors contributing to disease emergence.
Infection Control Procedures	Implement documented procedures in healthcare settings, including: - Thorough hand washing - Regular cleaning of medical equipment
Universal Adherence to Guidelines	Ensure all healthcare workers follow infection control guidelines to reduce nosocomial infections.
Fundamental Public Health Measures	Maintain and improve basic public health measures to prevent resurgence of controlled conditions.
Antibiotic Stewardship	Promote proper use of antibiotics to combat resistance and prevent misuse against viral infections.

CONCLUSION

In conclusion, the period from 2019 to 2023 has been marked by a multitude of viral disease outbreaks, both emerging and re-emerging, that have posed significant challenges to global public health. These outbreaks have underscored the ever-present threat of viral infections and the necessity for comprehensive preparedness and response strategies. The factors contributing to the emergence and rapid dissemination of these viral diseases are multifaceted, ranging from genetic reassortment events to changing human-animal interactions and the influence of globalization. The diverse clinical manifestations, transmission dynamics, and diagnostic hurdles associated with these viruses have highlighted the need for robust surveillance systems and continuous advancements in diagnostic capabilities. Furthermore, this period has emphasized the crucial role of effective infection control measures and non-pharmaceutical interventions, such as physical distancing and travel restrictions, in mitigating the spread of viral outbreaks. Additionally, the importance of robust healthcare systems with adequate resources, including trained personnel, essential equipment, and innovative clinical management strategies, has become increasingly evident. As we move forward, it is imperative that we apply the knowledge gained during this period to enhance our collective preparedness for future public health emergencies. By fostering international collaboration, investing in cutting-edge research, and implementing evidence-based strategies, we can strengthen our ability to respond effectively to viral disease outbreaks, ultimately safeguarding global health and well-being.

REFERENCES

[1]   Mourya D, Yadav P, Ullas PT, *et al*. Emerging/re-emerging viral diseases & new viruses on the Indian horizon. Indian J Med Res 2019; 149(4): 447-67.
       [http://dx.doi.org/10.4103/ijmr.IJMR_1239_18] [PMID: 31411169]

[2]   Wilson ME. Geography of infectious diseases. Infect Dis 2010; 1055.

[3]   Baker RE, Mahmud AS, Miller IF, *et al*. Infectious disease in an era of global change. Nat Rev Microbiol 2022; 20(4): 193-205.
       [http://dx.doi.org/10.1038/s41579-021-00639-z] [PMID: 34646006]

[4]   Sankaran N, Weiss RA. Viruses: impact on science and society. Encyclopedia of Virology. 2021: 671.

[5]   Evans AS. Viral infections of humans: epidemiology and control. Springer Science & Business Media 2013.

[6]   Network WHOGIPS. Evolution of H5N1 avian influenza viruses in Asia. Emerg Infect Dis 2005; 11(10): 1515-26.
       [http://dx.doi.org/10.3201/eid1110.050644] [PMID: 16318689]

[7]   Oaks SC Jr, Shope RE, Lederberg J. Emerging infections: microbial threats to health in the United States. National Academies Press 1992.

[8]   Lederberg J, Hamburg MA, Smolinski MS. Microbial threats to health: emergence, detection, and response. National Academies Press 2003.

[9]   Fukunaga R, Glaziou P, Harris JB, Date A, Floyd K, Kasaeva T. Epidemiology of tuberculosis and progress toward meeting global targets—worldwide, 2019. MMWR Morb Mortal Wkly Rep 2021; 70(12): 427-30.
       [http://dx.doi.org/10.15585/mmwr.mm7012a4] [PMID: 33764960]

[10] Daoud A, Laktineh A, Macrander C, Mushtaq A, Soubani AO. Pulmonary complications of influenza infection: a targeted narrative review. Postgrad Med 2019; 131(5): 299-308.
[http://dx.doi.org/10.1080/00325481.2019.1592400] [PMID: 30845866]

[11] Chung JR, Rolfes MA, Flannery B, *et al.* Effects of influenza vaccination in the United States during the 2018–2019 influenza season. Clin Infect Dis 2020; 71(8): e368-76.
[http://dx.doi.org/10.1093/cid/ciz1244] [PMID: 31905401]

[12] Randolph AG, Vaughn F, Sullivan R, *et al.* Critically ill children during the 2009-2010 influenza pandemic in the United States. Pediatrics 2011; 128(6): e1450-8.
[http://dx.doi.org/10.1542/peds.2011-0774] [PMID: 22065262]

[13] Yan J, Grantham M, Pantelic J, *et al.* Infectious virus in exhaled breath of symptomatic seasonal influenza cases from a college community. Proc Natl Acad Sci USA 2018; 115(5): 1081-6.
[http://dx.doi.org/10.1073/pnas.1716561115] [PMID: 29348203]

[14] Blachere FM, Lindsley WG, Weber AM, *et al.* Detection of an avian lineage influenza A(H7N2) virus in air and surface samples at a New York City feline quarantine facility. Influenza Other Respir Viruses 2018; 12(5): 613-22.
[http://dx.doi.org/10.1111/irv.12572] [PMID: 29768714]

[15] Lewis D. Is the coronavirus airborne? Experts can't agree. Nature 2020; 580(7802): 175.
[http://dx.doi.org/10.1038/d41586-020-00974-w] [PMID: 32242113]

[16] Van Doremalen N, Bushmaker T, Morris DH, *et al.* Aerosol and surface stability of SARS-CoV-2 as compared with SARS-CoV-1. N Engl J Med 2020; 382(16): 1564-7.
[http://dx.doi.org/10.1056/NEJMc2004973] [PMID: 32182409]

[17] Arnold FW, Fuqua JL. Viral respiratory infections: a cause of community-acquired pneumonia or a predisposing factor? Curr Opin Pulm Med 2020; 26(3): 208-14.
[http://dx.doi.org/10.1097/MCP.0000000000000666] [PMID: 32068577]

[18] Varga Z, Flammer AJ, Steiger P, *et al.* Endothelial cell infection and endotheliitis in COVID-19. Lancet 2020; 395(10234): 1417-8.
[http://dx.doi.org/10.1016/S0140-6736(20)30937-5] [PMID: 32325026]

[19] Jain S, Self WH, Wunderink RG, *et al.* Community-acquired pneumonia requiring hospitalization among US adults. N Engl J Med 2015; 373(5): 415-27.
[http://dx.doi.org/10.1056/NEJMoa1500245] [PMID: 26172429]

[20] Jain S, Williams DJ, Arnold SR, *et al.* Community-acquired pneumonia requiring hospitalization among U.S. children. N Engl J Med 2015; 372(9): 835-45.
[http://dx.doi.org/10.1056/NEJMoa1405870] [PMID: 25714161]

[21] Saha S, Chadha M, Al Mamun A, *et al.* Influenza seasonality and vaccination timing in tropical and subtropical areas of southern and south-eastern Asia. Bull World Health Organ 2014; 92(5): 318-30.
[http://dx.doi.org/10.2471/BLT.13.124412] [PMID: 24839321]

[22] Chadha MS, Potdar VA, Saha S, *et al.* Dynamics of influenza seasonality at sub-regional levels in India and implications for vaccination timing. PLoS One 2015; 10(5): e0124122.
[http://dx.doi.org/10.1371/journal.pone.0124122] [PMID: 25938466]

[23] Garg G, Garg S, Kamal R, Das B, Singh A. The risk of crimean congo haemorrhagic fever in india as a growing health concern. Infect Disord Drug Targets 2024; 24(8): e180324228044.
[http://dx.doi.org/10.2174/0118715265281694240223113930]

[24] Alexander EC, Deep A. Characterization of a hepatitis outbreak in children, 2021 to 2022. JAMA Network Open. 2022; 5(10): e2237091.

[25] Garg S, Garg G, Singh A. The Resurgence of H3N2 in India: Is it Life-threatening? Curr Drug Targets 2023; 24(12): 931-3.
[http://dx.doi.org/10.2174/1389450124666230821092330] [PMID: 37605425]

[26]   Dissanayake HA, Seneviratne SL. Liver involvement in dengue viral infections. Rev Med Virol 2018; 28(2): e1971.
[http://dx.doi.org/10.1002/rmv.1971] [PMID: 29465794]

[27]   Itha S, Kashyap R, Krishnani N, Saraswat VA, Choudhuri G, Aggarwal R. Profile of liver involvement in dengue virus infection. Natl Med J India 2005; 18(3): 127-30.
[PMID: 16130612]

[28]   Mahmood R, Benzadid MS, Weston S, *et al.* Dengue outbreak 2019: clinical and laboratory profiles of dengue virus infection in Dhaka city. Heliyon 2021; 7(6): e07183.
[http://dx.doi.org/10.1016/j.heliyon.2021.e07183] [PMID: 34141938]

[29]   Razavi H. Global epidemiology of viral hepatitis. Gastroenterol Clin North Am 2020; 49(2): 179-89.
[http://dx.doi.org/10.1016/j.gtc.2020.01.001] [PMID: 32389357]

[30]   Suk-Fong Lok A. Hepatitis B treatment: what we know now and what remains to be researched. Hepatol Commun 2019; 3(1): 8-19.
[http://dx.doi.org/10.1002/hep4.1281] [PMID: 30619990]

[31]   Omosigho PO, John OO, Adigun OA, Hassan HK, Olabode ON, Micheal AS. The Re-emergence of Diphtheria Amidst Multiple Outbreaks in Nigeria. Infectious Disorders-Drug Targets (Formerly Current Drug Targets-Infectious Disorders). 2024; 24(4): 20-8.
[http://dx.doi.org/10.2174/0118715265251299231117045940]

[32]   Ashshi AM. The prevalence of dengue virus serotypes in asymptomatic blood donors reveals the emergence of serotype 4 in Saudi Arabia. Virol J 2017; 14(1): 107.
[http://dx.doi.org/10.1186/s12985-017-0768-7] [PMID: 28599678]

[33]   Chiu CY, Bres V, Yu G, *et al.* Genomic assays for identification of chikungunya virus in blood donors, Puerto Rico, 2014. Emerg Infect Dis 2015; 21(8): 1409-13.
[http://dx.doi.org/10.3201/eid2108.150458] [PMID: 26196378]

[34]   Beau F, Lastère S, Mallet HP, Mauguin S, Broult J, Laperche S. Impact on blood safety of the last arboviruses outbreaks in French Polynesia (2012–2018). Transfus Clin Biol 2020; 27(1): 4-9.
[http://dx.doi.org/10.1016/j.tracli.2019.12.001] [PMID: 31889619]

[35]   Arya SC, Agarwal N. Rapid point–of–care diagnosis of chikungunya virus infection. Asian Pac J Trop Dis 2011; 1(3): 230-1.
[http://dx.doi.org/10.1016/S2222-1808(11)60035-2]

[36]   Giménez-Richarte Á, de Salazar MO, Arbona C, *et al.* Prevalence of Chikungunya, Dengue and Zika viruses in blood donors: a systematic literature review and meta-analysis. Blood Transfus 2022; 20(4): 267-80.
[PMID: 34694219]

[37]   Borges L, Pithon-Curi TC, Curi R, Hatanaka E. COVID-19 and neutrophils: the relationship between hyperinflammation and neutrophil extracellular traps. Mediators of inflammation. 2020; 2020.

[38]   Wang H, Tang X, Fan H, *et al.* Potential mechanisms of hemorrhagic stroke in elderly COVID-19 patients. Aging (Albany NY) 2020; 12(11): 10022-34.
[http://dx.doi.org/10.18632/aging.103335] [PMID: 32527987]

[39]   Ray MS, Patel V, Raval A, *et al.* Management of giant amoebic liver abscess with severe sepsis by open drainage: a study of 28 cases in 20 years. International Surgery Journal 2023; 10(6): 1024-30.
[http://dx.doi.org/10.18203/2349-2902.isj20231729]

[40]   Zhang Q-F, Cui J-M, Huang X-J, *et al.* Morphology and morphogenesis of severe acute respiratory syndrome (SARS)-associated virus. Sheng Wu Hua Xue Yu Sheng Wu Wu Li Xue Bao (Shanghai) 2003; 35(6): 587-91.
[PMID: 12796822]

[41]   Gu JiAng GJ, Gong EnCong GE, Zhang Bo ZB, Zheng Jie ZJ, Gao ZiFen GZ, Zhong YanFeng ZY.

Multiple organ infection and the pathogenesis of SARS. 2005.

[42]   Fisman DN. Hemophagocytic syndromes and infection. Emerg Infect Dis 2000; 6(6): 601-8.
[http://dx.doi.org/10.3201/eid0606.000608] [PMID: 11076718]

[43]   Zhan J, Deng R, Tang J, *et al.* The spleen as a target in severe acute respiratory syndrome. FASEB J 2006; 20(13): 2321-8.
[http://dx.doi.org/10.1096/fj.06-6324com] [PMID: 17077309]

[44]   Omosigho PO, John OO, Olabode ON, Onyemaechi EE, Singh A. Dengue virus in africa; what to know about the virus? Journal of Applied Health Sciences and Medicine 2023; 3(3): 23-9.
[http://dx.doi.org/10.58614/jahsm332]

[45]   Simons-Linares CR, Imam Z, Chahal P. Viral-attributed acute pancreatitis: a systematic review. Dig Dis Sci 2021; 66(7): 2162-72.
[http://dx.doi.org/10.1007/s10620-020-06531-9] [PMID: 32789532]

[46]   Banks PA, Freeman ML. Gastroenterology PPCotACo. Practice guidelines in acute pancreatitis. Official journal of the American College of Gastroenterology| ACG. 2006; 101(10): 2379-400.

[47]   Prinz RA. Mechanisms of acute pancreatitis. Int J Pancreatol 1991; 9(1): 31-8.
[http://dx.doi.org/10.1007/BF02925576] [PMID: 1744444]

[48]   Sahoo S, Narang RK, Singh A. The marburg virus outbreak in west africa. Curr Drug Targets 2023; 24(5): 380-1.
[http://dx.doi.org/10.2174/1389450124666230213154319] [PMID: 36788691]

[49]   Carrillo-Hernández MY, Ruiz-Saenz J, Martínez-Gutiérrez M. Coinfection of Zika with Dengue and Chikungunya virus Zika Virus Biology, Transmission, and Pathology. Elsevier 2021; pp. 117-27.
[http://dx.doi.org/10.1016/B978-0-12-820268-5.00011-0]

[50]   Vareille M, Kieninger E, Edwards MR, Regamey N. The airway epithelium: soldier in the fight against respiratory viruses. Clin Microbiol Rev 2011; 24(1): 210-29.
[http://dx.doi.org/10.1128/CMR.00014-10] [PMID: 21233513]

[51]   Jegaskanda S, Reading PC, Kent SJ. Influenza-specific antibody-dependent cellular cytotoxicity: toward a universal influenza vaccine. J Immunol 2014; 193(2): 469-75.
[http://dx.doi.org/10.4049/jimmunol.1400432] [PMID: 24994909]

[52]   Ong CWM, Elkington PT, Friedland JS. Tuberculosis, pulmonary cavitation, and matrix metalloproteinases. Am J Respir Crit Care Med 2014; 190(1): 9-18.
[http://dx.doi.org/10.1164/rccm.201311-2106PP] [PMID: 24713029]

[53]   Chiu C, Openshaw PJ. Antiviral B cell and T cell immunity in the lungs. Nat Immunol 2015; 16(1): 18-26.
[http://dx.doi.org/10.1038/ni.3056] [PMID: 25521681]

[54]   Openshaw PJ, Chiu C. Protective and dysregulated T cell immunity in RSV infection. Curr Opin Virol 2013; 3(4): 468-74.
[http://dx.doi.org/10.1016/j.coviro.2013.05.005] [PMID: 23806514]

[55]   Krishnamoorthy N, Khare A, Oriss TB, *et al.* Early infection with respiratory syncytial virus impairs regulatory T cell function and increases susceptibility to allergic asthma. Nat Med 2012; 18(10): 1525-30.
[http://dx.doi.org/10.1038/nm.2896] [PMID: 22961107]

[56]   Abril-Rodriguez G, Ribas A. SnapShot: immune checkpoint inhibitors. Cancer cell. 2017; 31(6): 848, e1.
[http://dx.doi.org/10.1016/j.ccell.2017.05.010]

[57]   Simon AK, Hollander GA, McMichael A. Evolution of the immune system in humans from infancy to old age. Proceedings of the Royal Society B: Biological Sciences. 2015; 282(1821): 2014-3085.
[http://dx.doi.org/10.1098/rspb.2014.3085]

[58]   Olin A, Henckel E, Chen Y, Lakshmikanth T, Pou C, Mikes J. Stereotypic immune system development in newborn children. Cell. 2018; 174(5): 1277-92.
[http://dx.doi.org/10.1016/j.cell.2018.06.045]

[59]   Chackerian AA, Alt JM, Perera TV, Dascher CC, Behar SM. Dissemination of Mycobacterium tuberculosis is influenced by host factors and precedes the initiation of T-cell immunity. Infect Immun 2002; 70(8): 4501-9.
[http://dx.doi.org/10.1128/IAI.70.8.4501-4509.2002] [PMID: 12117962]

[60]   Wolf AJ, Desvignes L, Linas B, *et al.* Initiation of the adaptive immune response to *Mycobacterium tuberculosis* depends on antigen production in the local lymph node, not the lungs. J Exp Med 2008; 205(1): 105-15.
[http://dx.doi.org/10.1084/jem.20071367] [PMID: 18158321]

[61]   Reiley WW, Calayag MD, Wittmer ST, *et al.* ESAT-6-specific CD4 T cell responses to aerosol *Mycobacterium tuberculosis* infection are initiated in the mediastinal lymph nodes. Proc Natl Acad Sci USA 2008; 105(31): 10961-6.
[http://dx.doi.org/10.1073/pnas.0801496105] [PMID: 18667699]

[62]   Kumar A, Farhana A, Guidry L, Saini V, Hondalus M, Steyn AJC. Redox homeostasis in mycobacteria: the key to tuberculosis control? Expert Rev Mol Med 2011; 13: e39.
[http://dx.doi.org/10.1017/S1462399411002079] [PMID: 22172201]

[63]   Ong CWM, Fox K, Ettorre A, Elkington PT, Friedland JS. Hypoxia increases neutrophil-driven matrix destruction after exposure to Mycobacterium tuberculosis. Sci Rep 2018; 8(1): 11475.
[http://dx.doi.org/10.1038/s41598-018-29659-1] [PMID: 30065292]

[64]   Lin PL, Flynn JL, Eds. CD8 T cells and Mycobacterium tuberculosis infection Seminars in immunopathology. Springer 2015.

[65]   Chan J, Mehta S, Bharrhan S, Chen Y, Achkar JM, Casadevall A, Eds. The role of B cells and humoral immunity in Mycobacterium tuberculosis infection Seminars in immunology. Elsevier 2014.

[66]   Day CL, Abrahams DA, Lerumo L, *et al.* Functional capacity of Mycobacterium tuberculosis-specific T cell responses in humans is associated with mycobacterial load. J Immunol 2011; 187(5): 2222-32.
[http://dx.doi.org/10.4049/jimmunol.1101122] [PMID: 21775682]

[67]   Day CL, Moshi ND, Abrahams DA, *et al.* Patients with tuberculosis disease have Mycobacterium tuberculosis-specific CD8 T cells with a pro-apoptotic phenotype and impaired proliferative capacity, which is not restored following treatment. PLoS One 2014; 9(4): e94949.
[http://dx.doi.org/10.1371/journal.pone.0094949] [PMID: 24740417]

[68]   Chiacchio RGD, Prioste FES, Vanstreels RET, *et al.* Health evaluation and survey of zoonotic pathogens in free-ranging capybaras (Hydrochoerus hydrochaeris). J Wildl Dis 2014; 50(3): 496-504.
[http://dx.doi.org/10.7589/2013-05-109] [PMID: 24779462]

[69]   Pinsky BA, Hayden RT. Cost-effective respiratory virus testing. J Clin Microbiol 2019; 57(9): e00373-19.
[http://dx.doi.org/10.1128/JCM.00373-19] [PMID: 31142607]

[70]   Almekhlafi GA, Albarrak MM, Mandourah Y, *et al.* Presentation and outcome of Middle East respiratory syndrome in Saudi intensive care unit patients. Crit Care 2016; 20(1): 123.
[http://dx.doi.org/10.1186/s13054-016-1303-8] [PMID: 27153800]

[71]   Midgley CM, Jackson MA, Selvarangan R, Turabelidze G, Obringer E, Johnson D. Severe respiratory illness associated with enterovirus D68—Missouri and Illinois. Elsevier 2014; pp. 2662-3.

[72]   Zhu N, Zhang D, Wang W, *et al.* A novel coronavirus from patients with pneumonia in China, 2019. N Engl J Med 2020; 382(8): 727-33.
[http://dx.doi.org/10.1056/NEJMoa2001017] [PMID: 31978945]

[73]   Wumkes ML, van der Velden AMT, de Bruin E, *et al.* Microarray profile of the humoral immune

response to influenza vaccination in breast cancer patients treated with chemotherapy. Vaccine 2017; 35(9): 1299-305.
[http://dx.doi.org/10.1016/j.vaccine.2017.01.039] [PMID: 28169075]

[74]   Goodwin S, McPherson JD, McCombie WR. Coming of age: ten years of next-generation sequencing technologies. Nat Rev Genet 2016; 17(6): 333-51.
[http://dx.doi.org/10.1038/nrg.2016.49] [PMID: 27184599]

[75]   Li CX, Li W, Zhou J, *et al*. High resolution metagenomic characterization of complex infectomes in paediatric acute respiratory infection. Sci Rep 2020; 10(1): 3963.
[http://dx.doi.org/10.1038/s41598-020-60992-6] [PMID: 32127629]

[76]   Kufner V, Plate A, Schmutz S, *et al*. Two years of viral metagenomics in a tertiary diagnostics unit: evaluation of the first 105 cases. Genes (Basel) 2019; 10(9): 661.
[http://dx.doi.org/10.3390/genes10090661] [PMID: 31470675]

[77]   Gillim-Ross L, Subbarao K. Emerging respiratory viruses: challenges and vaccine strategies. Clin Microbiol Rev 2006; 19(4): 614-36.
[http://dx.doi.org/10.1128/CMR.00005-06] [PMID: 17041137]

[78]   Regmi K, Lwin CM. Factors associated with the implementation of non-pharmaceutical interventions for reducing coronavirus disease 2019 (COVID-19): A systematic review. Int J Environ Res Public Health 2021; 18(8): 4274.
[http://dx.doi.org/10.3390/ijerph18084274] [PMID: 33920613]

[79]   Organization WH. WHO guidelines on the use of vaccines and antivirals during influenza pandemics. World Health Organization 2004.

[80]   Hatchett RJ, Mecher CE, Lipsitch M. Public health interventions and epidemic intensity during the 1918 influenza pandemic. Proc Natl Acad Sci USA 2007; 104(18): 7582-7.
[http://dx.doi.org/10.1073/pnas.0610941104] [PMID: 17416679]

[81]   Migliori GB, Nardell E, Yedilbayev A, *et al*. Reducing tuberculosis transmission: a consensus document from the World Health Organization Regional Office for Europe. Eur Respir J 2019; 53(6): 1900391.
[http://dx.doi.org/10.1183/13993003.00391-2019] [PMID: 31023852]

[82]   Thorne CD, Khozin S, McDiarmid MA. Using the hierarchy of control technologies to improve healthcare facility infection control: lessons from severe acute respiratory syndrome. J Occup Environ Med 2004; 46(7): 613-22.
[http://dx.doi.org/10.1097/01.jom.0000134191.92225.f2] [PMID: 15247800]

[83]   Leung CC, Lam TH, Cheng KK. Mass masking in the COVID-19 epidemic: people need guidance. Lancet 2020; 395(10228): 945.
[http://dx.doi.org/10.1016/S0140-6736(20)30520-1] [PMID: 32142626]

[84]   Leung CC, Lam TH, Cheng KK. Let us not forget the mask in our attempts to stall the spread of COVID-19. Int J Tuberc Lung Dis 2020; 24(4): 364-6.
[http://dx.doi.org/10.5588/ijtld.20.0124] [PMID: 32317058]

[85]   MacIntyre CR, Seale H, Dung TC, *et al*. A cluster randomised trial of cloth masks compared with medical masks in healthcare workers. BMJ Open 2015; 5(4): e006577.
[http://dx.doi.org/10.1136/bmjopen-2014-006577] [PMID: 25903751]

[86]   Esposito S, Principi N, Leung CC, Migliori GB. Universal use of face masks for success against COVID-19: evidence and implications for prevention policies. Eur Respir J 2020; 55(6): 2001260.
[http://dx.doi.org/10.1183/13993003.01260-2020] [PMID: 32350103]

[87]   Hong LX, Lin A, He ZB, *et al*. Mask wearing in pre-symptomatic patients prevents SARS-CoV-2 transmission: An epidemiological analysis. Travel Med Infect Dis 2020; 36: 101803.
[http://dx.doi.org/10.1016/j.tmaid.2020.101803] [PMID: 32592903]

[88]   Organization WH. Modes of transmission of virus causing COVID-19: implications for IPC

precaution recommendations: scientific brief, 29 March 2020. World Health Organization 2020.

[89]   Lai MYY, Cheng PKC, Lim WWL. Survival of severe acute respiratory syndrome coronavirus. Clin Infect Dis 2005; 41(7): e67-71.
[http://dx.doi.org/10.1086/433186] [PMID: 16142653]

[90]   Rabenau HF, Cinatl J, Morgenstern B, Bauer G, Preiser W, Doerr HW. Stability and inactivation of SARS coronavirus. Med Microbiol Immunol (Berl) 2005; 194(1-2): 1-6.
[http://dx.doi.org/10.1007/s00430-004-0219-0] [PMID: 15118911]

[91]   Wong JCC, Hapuarachchi HC, Arivalan S, *et al.* Environmental contamination of SARS-CoV-2 in a non-healthcare setting. Int J Environ Res Public Health 2020; 18(1): 117.
[http://dx.doi.org/10.3390/ijerph18010117] [PMID: 33375308]

[92]   Berger A, Drosten C, Doerr HW, Stürmer M, Preiser W. Severe acute respiratory syndrome (SARS)—paradigm of an emerging viral infection. J Clin Virol 2004; 29(1): 13-22.
[http://dx.doi.org/10.1016/j.jcv.2003.09.011] [PMID: 14675864]

[93]   Bonny TS, Yezli S, Lednicky JA. Isolation and identification of human coronavirus 229E from frequently touched environmental surfaces of a university classroom that is cleaned daily. Am J Infect Control 2018; 46(1): 105-7.
[http://dx.doi.org/10.1016/j.ajic.2017.07.014] [PMID: 28893443]

[94]   Dara M, Sotgiu G, Reichler MR, Chiang C-Y, Chee CBE, Migliori GB. New diseases and old threats: lessons from tuberculosis for the COVID-19 response. Int J Tuberc Lung Dis 2020; 24(5): 544-5.
[http://dx.doi.org/10.5588/ijtld.20.0151] [PMID: 32398212]

[95]   McKee M, Stuckler D. If the world fails to protect the economy, COVID-19 will damage health not just now but also in the future. Nat Med 2020; 26(5): 640-2.
[http://dx.doi.org/10.1038/s41591-020-0863-y] [PMID: 32273610]

[96]   Organization WH. COVID-19 strategic preparedness and response plan: monitoring and evaluation framework, 11 May 2021. World Health Organization 2021.

[97]   Qian X, Ren R, Wang Y, *et al.* Fighting against the common enemy of COVID-19: a practice of building a community with a shared future for mankind. Infect Dis Poverty 2020; 9(1): 34.
[http://dx.doi.org/10.1186/s40249-020-00650-1] [PMID: 32264957]

[98]   Pathirathna R, Adikari P, Dias D, Gunathilake U. Critical preparedness, readiness, and responses to the covid-19 pandemic: A narrative. Jurnal Administrasi Kesehatan Indonesia Vol. 2020; 8(1).

[99]   Smith AC, Thomas E, Snoswell CL, *et al.* Telehealth for global emergencies: Implications for coronavirus disease 2019 (COVID-19). J Telemed Telecare 2020; 26(5): 309-13.
[http://dx.doi.org/10.1177/1357633X20916567] [PMID: 32196391]

[100]   Canestrini N. Covid-19 Italian emergency legislation and infection of the rule of law. New Journal of European Criminal Law 2020; 11(2): 116-22.
[http://dx.doi.org/10.1177/2032284420934669]

CHAPTER 2

Outbreak of SARS-CoV-2 (COVID-19)

Prabhjot Kaur[1], Anish Soni[2], Pawan Kumar[1], Bharat Sharma[2], Prabhjot Kaur[3], Rohit Bhatia[1], Subramanya Sarma Ganti[1] and Naresh Kumar Rangra[4,*]

[1] *Department of Pharmaceutical Chemistry, ISF College of Pharmacy, Moga, Punjab-142001, India*

[2] *Department of Pharmaceutical Analysis, ISF College of Pharmacy, Moga, Punjab-142001, India*

[3] *Department of Food and Nutrition, Punjab Agricultural University, Ludhiana, Punjab-141004, India*

[4] *Chitkara University School of Pharmacy, Chitkara University, Baddi, Himachal Pradesh, India*

Abstract: First detected in late 2019, the SARS-CoV-2 virus quickly became a worldwide public health issue. This publication offers a thorough analysis of COVID-19's traits, features, modes of transmission, available treatments, prevalence, case studies, and World Health Organization (WHO) recommendations. The recently emerged coronavirus, SARS-CoV-2, has unique proteins and genetic material that echo those seen in the earlier outbreaks of SARS and MERS. It addresses how the disease can spread through a variety of channels, including sexual, ocular, fecal-oral, respiratory, indirect, and vertical. Effective treatment techniques, such as antiviral medicines, immunomodulatory treatments, traditional Chinese medicine, and targeted immunotherapy approaches, are presented. People with COVID-19 experience a spectrum of illnesses, from feeling slightly unwell to becoming critically sick. There have been millions of confirmed cases and fatalities from COVID-19 worldwide, marking unprecedented levels of prevalence. The advent of the JN.1 variety is one of the recent events that highlight the virus's dynamic character and the significance of continued study and public health initiatives. The World Health Organization has recommended that vaccination, physical separation, mask use, hand hygiene, and early medical attention be prioritized as essential tactics to reduce the spread of the pandemic and manage it. This publication aims to be a weapon in the fight against COVID-19, providing in-depth knowledge about the virus.

Keywords: Coronavirus, Genomic features, JN.1 variant, Pandemic, Structural proteins, SARS-CoV-2, WHO recommendations.

---

* Corresponding author Naresh Kumar Rangra: Chitkara University School of Pharmacy, Chitkara University, Baddi, Himachal Pradesh, India; E-mail: nareshrangra@gmail.com

INTRODUCTION

SARS-CoV-2, a coronavirus, is the virus responsible for the respiratory illness COVID-19. It is a strain of the species that shares the same family as the virus that caused the SARS pandemic in 2002–2004. In late 2019, a highly contagious and pathogenic coronavirus surfaced, sparking the global COVID-19 pandemic. SARSCoV2, the novel coronavirus that causes the new COVID-19 disease, most likely started in Wuhan, China. The Wuhan health officials identified a few instances of atypical pneumonia in the middle of December 2019, which was subsequently caused by a new coronavirus. At the beginning of November 2019, it possibly transferred from an animal reservoir to a person [1]. Scientists traced the cause of the outbreak to an RNA virus. This virus belonged to the same family of coronaviruses as the ones responsible for the MERS pandemic in 2012 and the SARS pandemic in 2003 [2]. The SARS-CoV-2 virus has a simple strand of genetic material (RNA) that carries the instructions for building the spiky outer shell, envelope, membrane, and core of the virus. As of May 20, 2020, according to data from multiple sources, over 5,090,118 cases of COVID-19 have been reported worldwide, with more than 333,000 deaths. 2,546,198 people have recovered [3]. COVID-19 is spread by touch with open surfaces or by droplets released during speaking or sneezing within a 2-meter radius. Half of the transmissions happen due to coming into contact with an asymptomatic person. In fact, in asymptomatic patients without nasal obstruction, anosmia is a symptom of COVID-19 infection. Furthermore, the patient has up to two weeks after the disease's symptoms have subsided to spread the illness. It is said to be unlikely for fecal-oral stool to transmit. No evidence of perinatal transmission has been found [4]. Medical professionals, public health officials, academics, and media are finding it difficult to stay current with the copious and constantly changing quantity of knowledge regarding COVID-19. We performed a thorough literature review of the SARS-CoV-2 Virus and the Coronavirus Disease 2019 (COVID-19) to provide a clear understanding of the substantial material that is accessible, mentioning the characteristics, features, prevalence, no. of cases and treatment, and WHO recommendations in this chapter [5, 6].

Characteristics

A group of viruses called Coronaviridae belong to bigger groups, which are known as Nidovirales that contain coronaviruses, which infect humans and a wide range of other animals with disorders of the neurological, digestive, and respiratory systems. With a diameter of between 80 and 160 mm, coronavirus particles are spherically shaped [7]. The outer shell of the coronavirus has spike proteins. Beneath these spikes are envelope and membrane proteins, which form a protective layer. Inside this shell lies a coiled structure called the nucleocapsid.

This nucleocapsid is made up of RNA, the virus's genetic material, and proteins that bind to it [1, 2]. Compared to other RNA viruses, the coronavirus has a heavyweight genetic code. This single strand of information, ranging from 26,000 to 32,000 units long, carries the instructions for the virus. The coronavirus's genetic code is a complex set of instructions packed into a single strand of RNA. This code is divided into six sections, each containing the blueprint for a different viral component. It is like a recipe with specific sections for the ingredients and assembly instructions. Guaranteeing the code functions properly, special caps are attached to each end. Interestingly, the first part of the code contains instructions for 16 helper proteins crucial for making copies of the viral RNA. The remaining sections hold the code for the virus's building blocks: four proteins forming its outer shell and core, and eight additional proteins that play a vital role in assembling new virus particles [8 - 10]. Even though SARS-CoV-2 and SARS-CoV share many similarities in their protein structures and building blocks (amino acids), particularly in specific proteins like S, ORF8, ORF3b, and ORF10. They even share a similar code section (Orf1ab) for creating essential helper proteins and the standard four structural proteins found in coronaviruses. Despite these resemblances, there are also some key differences between the two viruses [11]. Researchers have produced copies of most SARS-CoV-2 proteins in human cells, revealing that a small protein, ORF10, shared some similarities with the same protein in the original SARS virus. Despite its size, ORF10 can latch onto a cellular disposal unit and disrupt its function, potentially aiding the virus in hijacking the cell. However, this cellular machine might also target ORF10 for destruction, hindering viral replication [12].

Routes of Transmission

The coronavirus is spread while sneezing, coughing respiratory droplets, and aerosols that are released when someone coughs or sneezes and land in the mouth, nose, or eyes of those nearby. Physically separating yourself from sick people by at least one meter greatly reduces this route of transmission, underscoring the significance of keeping a safe distance from them. Although short-range aerosols and respiratory droplets are thought to be the primary modes of transmission, longer-range aerosol transmission is also conceivable; some researchers have suggested dispersal distances of up to ten feet. Direct contact with sick individuals is still the greatest worry, although indirect transmission through contaminated surfaces is also a possible pathway. Simple preventive measures such as wearing a mask, avoiding crowded areas, and washing your hands often can reduce the chances of catching the coronavirus. However, the specific pathways of viral transmission are described here.

Respiratory Transmission

Similar to SARS and MERS viruses, COVID-19 caused by SARS-CoV-2 mainly affects the respiratory system. People infected typically experience fever, cough, and difficulty breathing. However, these symptoms are common in many lower respiratory tract infections and aren't specific enough to diagnose COVID-19 on their own [13].

Indirect Transmission

SARS-CoV-2 spreads *via* infected surfaces or items as opposed to direct person-to-person contact which is referred to as indirect transmission. The risk of transmission through fomites increases due to the virus's ability to persist alive and infectious on surfaces for prolonged periods, as demonstrated by studies. When dust particles or larger respiratory droplets evaporate and contain microorganisms in their droplet nuclei smaller than 5 μm in diameter, airborne transmission takes place. This enables bacteria to go farther than one meter and stay in the air for longer periods. When particles aerosolize, airborne transmission becomes dangerous, particularly during critical operations like cardiac resuscitation, bronchoscopy, and endotracheal intubation [14].

Fecal-oral Route of Transmission

Research has indicated that the possibility of fecal-oral transmission may stem from the ability of extended viral shedding in fecal matter. A case study revealed that an asymptomatic COVID-19 patient had positive results from the nasopharyngeal sample, but there was persistent viral identification in the faeces for up to 42 days [15].

Vertical Route of Transmission

There are different ways a mom could pass the SARS-CoV-2 virus (the virus that causes COVID-19) to her baby. This includes during pregnancy, childbirth, or even after birth while breastfeeding. This way of spreading the virus is called vertical transmission. Research has focused on the possibility of a mother transmitting the virus to her developing baby in the womb, which could lead to infection after birth. Studies have found elevated IgM antibodies in some babies born to mothers with COVID-19, raising the possibility that the virus might have passed from mother to child during pregnancy [16 - 18].

Sexual Route of Transmission

Researchers are examining whether COVID-19 (caused by the SARS-CoV-2 virus) can spread through sexual activity. While studies have not definitively proven it, they have found the virus in semen and some body fluids. This suggests sexual practices like anal or oral sex could be a potential route of transmission, though more research is needed. A recent study conducted by Li *et al.* tested semen samples from 38 men. Six samples (16%) came back positive for SARS-CoV-2. Interestingly, four of these positive results were from men experiencing the most severe symptoms, while the other two were from men who were recovering [19].

Ocular Route of Transmission

The possibility of the virus spreading through the eyes and ocular surfaces is known as the ocular mode of transmission of SARS-CoV-2. Research has demonstrated that SARS-CoV-2 may result in ocular problems. Ocular symptoms include conjunctival congestion, dry eye, blurred vision, and a feeling of a foreign body clinical manifestations were seen in patients infected by the coronavirus. According to research, the virus may reproduce in the conjunctiva and infect the eye, which raises worries about the likelihood of transmission through ocular fluid. While some researchers have reported finding viral RNA in conjunctival tissues, others have only found weak evidence of the presence of the virus. According to a case study, viral shedding happens in the eyes when COVID-19 presents inflammation in the eyes around two weeks after the start of the illness. The samples from the eyes were taken which confirms the presence of the virus [20].

Features

COVID-19 (caused by the SARS-CoV-2 virus) can cause a whole spectrum of symptoms, from barely noticeable to very serious [21 - 24] (Fig. **1**). According to studies, symptoms such as anosmia or ageusia are important markers of an active SARS-CoV-2 infection, particularly when combined with fever. Additionally, cough plays a crucial role in the diagnosis of COVID-19, especially when it is accompanied by shortness of breath and chest pain. Headache and diarrhea are two more less specific symptoms. It is noteworthy that certain individuals infected with SARS-CoV-2 may not exhibit any symptoms at all or only exhibit mild ones, underscoring the heterogeneity in the virus's presentation in various people. It is noteworthy that certain people do not show any symptoms while they are infected by the virus. The most common symptoms include:

- **Fever:** A fever is one of the most frequent signs of COVID-19. Generally, a temperature at or above 100.4°F (38°C) is considered a fever. Many people with COVID-19 experience a rise in body temperature to 38°C or even higher.
- **Cough:** Persistent cough, often dry, is a common symptom. It can range from mild to severe.

- **Shortness of Breath or Difficulty Breathing:** In case of severe cases, patients may face difficulty in breathing, which is a warning sign and this condition needs urgent medical help.
- **Fatigue:** Many people with COVID-19 report feeling tired or exhausted, even with minimal physical exertion.
- **Muscle or Body Aches:** Muscle pain, body aches, and general discomfort are common symptoms, similar to those experienced with the flu.
- **Headache:** Headaches, sometimes severe, can occur as a symptom of COVID-19.
- **Inability to Taste and Smell:** Loss of the sense of taste or smell is a distinctive symptom associated with SARS-CoV-2 infection.
- **Sore Throat:** A sore or scratchy throat is another symptom that can occur with COVID-19.
- **Chills:** Shivering or feeling cold despite having a fever is common.
- **Congestion or Runny Nose:** Common cold-like symptoms such as stuffy or runny nose are seen in patients infected by the virus.
- **Nausea or Vomiting:** Gastrointestinal symptoms, including nausea and vomiting, have been reported in some cases.
- **Diarrhea:** Digestive issues, such as diarrhea, may also occur in some individuals with COVID-19.

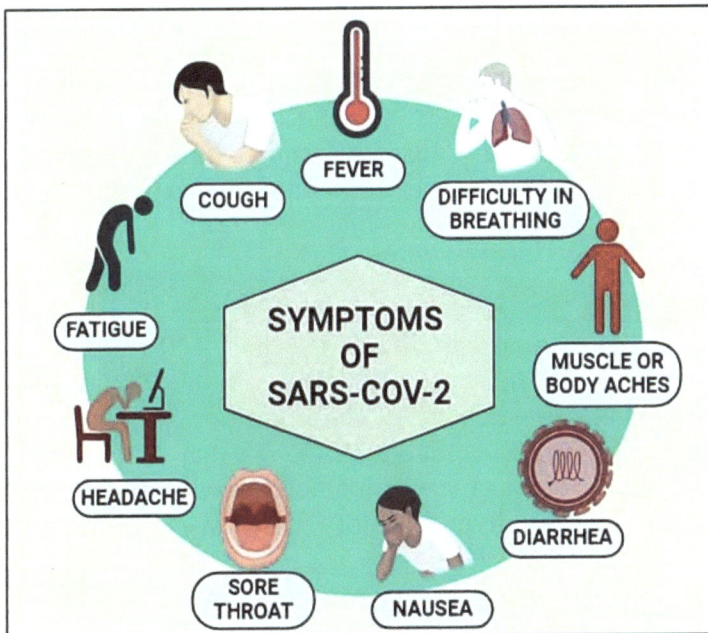

Fig. (1). Symptoms of SARS-COV-2.

It's vital to know that symptoms might emerge 2–14 days following contact with the virus. COVID-19 acts differently in everyone. Some people might not feel sick at all (asymptomatic), while others can get very sick. In severe cases, COVID-19 can cause pneumonia, acute respiratory distress syndrome (ARDS), and even death.

Treatment

During that time, there was a lot of discussion about COVID-19 therapy choices. With the support of foreign researchers, effective treatment methods were exchanged, improving the prognosis of COVID-19 patients. There were early hopes that treating COVID-19 patients with cell therapy and medications that boost the immune system (immunotherapy) could be helpful. Numerous therapeutic options were used, such as respiratory assistance for severe pulmonary difficulties, antiviral treatments for immunocompromised individuals or those who were at risk of developing severe forms of the disease, and symptomatic relief with medications such as paracetamol for pain or fever. RT-PCR and other virological assays were the most reliable means of confirming infection, underscoring the significance of early detection. Vaccination was the best line of defense against COVID-19 since it reduced the likelihood of transmission and serious illness. Booster doses were recommended to maintain protection over time, especially considering the established effectiveness of mRNA vaccines.

Using masks, washing your hands frequently, and coughing with the right technique were all crucial precautions to take to stop the transmission of SARS-CoV-2. Effective COVID-19 patient therapies based on recent research and/or Chinese experience were offered in this comprehensive description [25 - 28].

Chloroquine and Hydroxychloroquine

According to Chinese recommendations, chloroquine should be used in clinical therapy following a previous experiment in which 100 COVID-19 patients were proven to be able to suppress the virus. *In vitro*, studies showed that hydroxychloroquine, an analogue of chloroquine, had a greater degree of safety and a stronger inhibitory effect on SARS-CoV-2 than chloroquine. Furthermore, in persons with severe illness for which glucocorticoids and immunosuppressants are unsuccessful, low-dose hydroxychloroquine may have an immunoregulatory role and reduce the cytokine storm [29 - 31].

Immunomodulatory Therapy

The use of anakinra, tocilizumab, and dexamethasone for COVID-19 has received a lot of attention lately. 2100 COVID-19 patients were enrolled in a sizable

RECOVERY trial to assess the treatment efficacy of dexamethasone. Remarkably, it showed that in hospitalized patients with severe complications, dexamethasone could lower mortality by as much as 33%. Due to its significant impact on lowering COVID-19 patient mortality, dexamethasone—a readily accessible and inexpensive steroid—is anticipated to be a highly efficacious and reasonably priced therapy option. Tocilizumab, the first IL-6 receptor inhibitor, has a significant influence on the way COVID-19 patients are treated [32 - 34].

Traditional Chinese Medicine (TCM)

TCM improves symptoms and lowers COVID-19 worsening, death, and recurrence rates, all of which are favourable outcomes. TCM was utilized by 91.5% of COVID-19 patients in China, and its effectiveness was higher than 90%. According to research from China, TCM can influence ACE2 dysfunction brought on by viral infection through a variety of mechanisms. Additionally, it can prevent viral multiplication by inhibiting ribosomal proteins, which offers protection to people. Furthermore, by controlling Th17 and cytokine-related pathways, Traditional Chinese Medicine (TCM) might help COVID-19 patients by calming down an overactive immune system response. This could potentially protect patients from harm [35 - 37].

Specific Immunotherapy

Vaccination

Vaccines developed using adenovirus vectors, weakened influenza viruses, inactivated viruses, recombinant proteins, and nucleic acids (like mRNA and DNA) have all been part of the research efforts to combat COVID-19 [38, 39].

Passive Immunity

Monoclonal antibody injections are a useful treatment for viral infections as well as a means of preventing them in the short term. Monoclonal antibodies designed to fight SARS target a specific region (receptor-binding domain or RBD) of the S protein on the outer surface (envelope) of the SARS-CoV virus [40].

Cell Therapy

It is anticipated that cell therapy will become a new weapon in the fight against SARS-CoV-2; in fact, China has created programs on stem cell therapy for COVID-19 (ChiCTR2000030020). Because mesenchymal stem cells are located at the site of inflammation, they exert immunomodulatory actions that reduce inflammation and regulate cytokines linked to inflammation [41].

Prevalence

Since its emergence over three years ago, COVID-19 has wreaked havoc on a global scale. By January 7, 2024, a staggering 774.8 million confirmed cases and nearly 7.01 million deaths had been recorded worldwide (Fig. **2**).

Fig. (2). Nation-wise reported cases of SARS-CoV 2.

During this period, nearly every WHO region witnessed its worst outbreak since the pandemic began. Southeast Asia reached its peak in May 2021, while Europe, Africa, the Americas, and the Eastern Mediterranean saw a surge in cases concentrated between December 2021 and January 2022. As of March 2022, the Western Pacific region was experiencing the highest number of new cases, with some Pacific Island nations just starting to grapple with community spread of the virus. Between March 2022 and January 1st, 2023, there were roughly 656 million documented cases of COVID-19 worldwide, with around 6.6 million fatalities. (Fig. **3**), and from January 1st 2023 to January 7th, 2024, there has been an increase in SAR-CoV-2 cases, with reported infections reaching approximately 774 million globally, and fatalities rising to around 7 million during this period [42, 43].

Case Studies

At the end of 2019, the WHO China Country Office was alerted to pneumonia cases of unknown origin in Wuhan, China. By January 3, 2020, 44 cases were reported with an unidentified cause. On January 11 and 12, 2020, the WHO received information linking the outbreak to a seafood market in Wuhan. Chinese authorities identified a new coronavirus on January 7, and its genetic sequence was shared on January 12 for diagnostic kit development [44]. The spread of COVID-19 has been tremendous throughout the years, however, there have been several cases of this deadly virus within this period. Many people have recovered and unfortunately, the country has also witnessed many fatalities. Given below are the cases of COVID-19 from 2019- 2023 (Fig. **4**) [45].

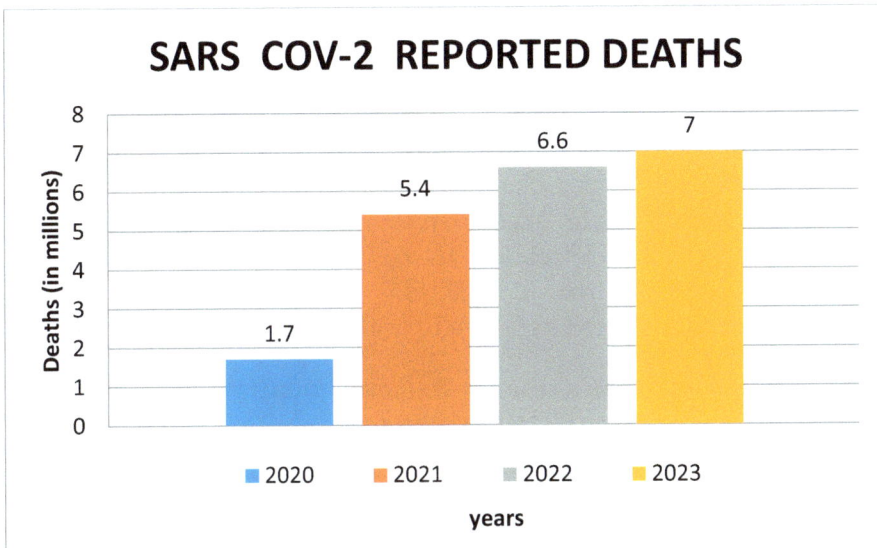

Fig. (3). Reported deaths per year (2019-2023).

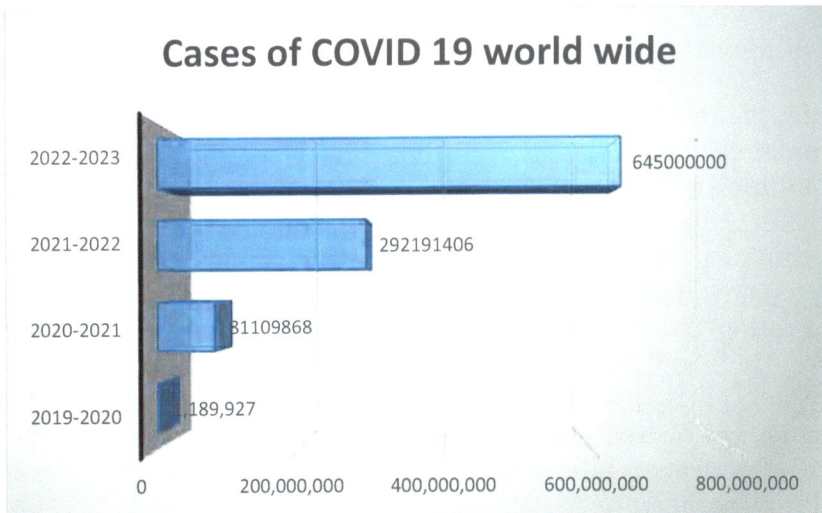

Fig. (4). Worldwide cases of COVID-19 from 2019-2023.

Recently a new outbreak in the world which is the JN. 1 variant has now turned into a global threat. Health authorities are concerned about the COVID-19 virus, which belongs to the Omicron family, and specifically targets the JN.1 variety was first identified in December 2023. It is distinguished by a unique alteration in its spike protein known as SL455S. This modification seems to make the virus more adept at eluding the immune system, which could account for why it spreads more readily than previous varieties [46]. The fact that JN.1 is displaying resistance to XBB.1.5, a specific kind of vaccine, is concerning because it calls into question how well our current vaccinations can protect against it. This virus mutation may alter the way the virus spreads and the efficacy of our vaccinations against it. It serves as a reminder that the virus is dynamic and that researchers are keeping a careful eye on these changes to modify our approaches to combat COVID-19. Data collected up to December 16, 2023 showed a significant rise in a particular strain of COVID-19 called JN.1. During epidemiological week 48 (from November 27 to December 3, 2023), JN.1 sequences made up 27.1% of all COVID-19 sequences submitted to GISAID from 41 countries worldwide [47].

WHO (World Health Organization) Recommendations or Advice for the Public: Coronavirus Disease (COVID-19)

Regarding the COVID-19 pandemic, there were several important rules that one must strictly follow to safeguard oneself and society as a whole. These guidelines encompass a range of practices that include following local vaccination recommendations, ensuring a minimum physical distance of at least one meter from others, steering clear of crowded and poorly ventilated spaces, wearing masks that fit properly in situations where maintaining distance is challenging, maintaining regular hand hygiene through washing with soap and water or using alcohol-based sanitizers, covering one's mouth and nose when sneezing or coughing, promptly self-isolating if feeling unwell or displaying COVID-19 symptoms, ensuring masks cover the mouth, nose, and chin adequately, opting for outdoor gatherings whenever feasible, improving indoor ventilation to reduce the risk of transmission, upholding good respiratory etiquette, seeking medical assistance promptly if experiencing symptoms like fever, cough, or difficulty breathing, wearing a mask when outside the home and self-isolating for a specified period if unwell, and staying informed by accessing updates from reputable sources such as the World Health Organization and local health agencies. To protect oneself and aid in the overall effort to stop the virus from spreading, it is critical to follow the recommendations given by regional and federal health authorities [48 - 50].

CONCLUSION

The COVID-19 pandemic caused by the SARS-CoV-2 virus has been an unprecedented global health crisis. This comprehensive chapter has provided an in-depth analysis of various aspects of the virus and disease, including its characteristics, modes of transmission, features, treatment options, prevalence data, case studies, and recommendations from the World Health Organization. The highly contagious and pathogenic nature of SARS-CoV-2, coupled with its ability to undergo mutations, has made it a formidable challenge for healthcare systems and societies worldwide. The chapter has highlighted the diverse symptoms of COVID-19, ranging from asymptomatic cases to severe respiratory distress, underscoring the heterogeneity of the disease's presentation. While significant progress has been made in developing effective treatments, such as antivirals, immunomodulatory therapies, and vaccines, the emergence of new variants like JN.1 serves as a reminder that the battle against COVID-19 is ongoing. Continuous research, vigilance, and adaptation of strategies are crucial to mitigating the impact of the virus.

The WHO's recommendations, emphasizing vaccination, physical distancing, mask-wearing, hand hygiene, and early medical attention, remain pivotal in controlling the spread of the pandemic. Collective efforts and adherence to these guidelines are essential for protecting individuals and communities. Looking ahead, this chapter serves as a comprehensive resource and a call to action, highlighting the importance of preparedness, global cooperation, and sustained efforts to combat the COVID-19 pandemic and future infectious disease threats. By learning from the experiences and insights shared in this work, we can better navigate the challenges posed by emerging viral pathogens and safeguard public health on a global scale.

REFERENCES

[1]   Domingo JL. What we know and what we need to know about the origin of SARS-CoV-2. Environ Res 2021; 200: 111785.
[http://dx.doi.org/10.1016/j.envres.2021.111785] [PMID: 34329631]

[2]   Lu R, Zhao X, Li J, *et al.* Genomic characterisation and epidemiology of 2019 novel coronavirus: implications for virus origins and receptor binding. Lancet 2020; 395(10224): 565-74.
[http://dx.doi.org/10.1016/S0140-6736(20)30251-8] [PMID: 32007145]

[3]   Simbana-Rivera K, Gomez-Barreno L, Guerrero J, Simbana-Guaycha F, Fernandez R, LopezCortes A. Interim analysis of pandemic Coronavirus Disease 2019; medRxiv 2020.04.25.20079863.

[4]   Peiris JSM, Guan Y, Yuen KY. Severe acute respiratory syndrome. Nat Med 2004; 10(S12) (Suppl.): S88-97.
[http://dx.doi.org/10.1038/nm1143] [PMID: 15577937]

[5]   Harapan H, Itoh N, Yufika A, *et al.* Coronavirus disease 2019 (COVID-19): A literature review. J Infect Public Health 2020; 13(5): 667-73.
[http://dx.doi.org/10.1016/j.jiph.2020.03.019] [PMID: 32340833]

[6]   Di Nardo M, van Leeuwen G, Loreti A, *et al.* A literature review of 2019 novel coronavirus (SARS-CoV2) infection in neonates and children. Pediatr Res 2021; 89(5): 1101-8.
[http://dx.doi.org/10.1038/s41390-020-1065-5] [PMID: 32679582]

[7]   Hu B, Guo H, Zhou P, Shi ZL. Characteristics of SARS-CoV-2 and COVID-19. Nat Rev Microbiol 2021; 19(3): 141-54.
[http://dx.doi.org/10.1038/s41579-020-00459-7] [PMID: 33024307]

[8]   Li G, Fan Y, Lai Y, *et al.* Coronavirus infections and immune responses. J Med Virol 2020; 92(4): 424-32.
[http://dx.doi.org/10.1002/jmv.25685] [PMID: 31981224]

[9]   Jin Y, Yang H, Ji W, *et al.* Virology, epidemiology, pathogenesis, and control of COVID-19. Viruses 2020; 12(4): 372.
[http://dx.doi.org/10.3390/v12040372] [PMID: 32230900]

[10]   Lu R, Zhao X, Li J, *et al.* Genomic characterisation and epidemiology of novel 2019.

[11]   Hoffmann M, Kleine-Weber H, Schroeder S, *et al.* SARS-CoV-2 cell entry depends on ace2 and tmprss2 and is blocked by a clinically proven protease inhibitor. Cell 2020; 181(2): 271-280.e8.
[http://dx.doi.org/10.1016/j.cell.2020.02.052] [PMID: 32142651]

[12]   Gordon DE, Jang GM, Bouhaddou M, *et al.* A SARS-CoV-2 protein interaction map reveals targets for drug repurposing. Nature 2020; 583(7816): 459-68.
[http://dx.doi.org/10.1038/s41586-020-2286-9] [PMID: 32353859]

[13]   Wu YC, Chen CS, Chan YJ. The outbreak of COVID-19: An overview. J Chin Med Assoc 2020; 83(3): 217-20.
[http://dx.doi.org/10.1097/JCMA.0000000000000270] [PMID: 32134861]

[14]   Modes of transmission of virus causing COVID-19: implications for IPC precaution recommendations: scientific brief, 27 March 2020. Retrieved from https://apps.who.int/iris/handle/10665/331601

[15]   Jiang X, Luo M, Zou Z, Wang X, Chen C, Qiu J. Asymptomatic SARS-CoV-2 infected case with viral detection positive in stool but negative in nasopharyngeal samples lasts for 42 days. J Med Virol 2020; 92(10): 1807-9.
[http://dx.doi.org/10.1002/jmv.25941] [PMID: 32330309]

[16]   Kimberlin DW, Stagno S. Can SARS-CoV-2 infection be acquired in utero?: more definitive evidence is needed. JAMA 2020; 323(18): 1788-9.
[http://dx.doi.org/10.1001/jama.2020.4868] [PMID: 32215579]

[17]   Dong L, Tian J, He S, *et al.* Possible vertical transmission of SARS-CoV-2 from an infected mother to her newborn. JAMA 2020; 323(18): 1846-8.
[http://dx.doi.org/10.1001/jama.2020.4621] [PMID: 32215581]

[18]   Zeng H, Xu C, Fan J, *et al.* Antibodies in infants born to mothers with COVID-19 pneumonia. JAMA 2020; 323(18): 1848-9.
[http://dx.doi.org/10.1001/jama.2020.4861] [PMID: 32215589]

[19]   Li D, Jin M, Bao P, Zhao W, Zhang S. Clinical characteristics and results of semen tests among men with coronavirus disease 2019. JAMA Netw Open 2020; 3(5): e208292-2.
[http://dx.doi.org/10.1001/jamanetworkopen.2020.8292] [PMID: 32379329]

[20]   Chen L, Liu M, Zhang Z, *et al.* Ocular manifestations of a hospitalised patient with confirmed 2019 novel coronavirus disease. Br J Ophthalmol, bjophthalmol, 2020; 316304.
[http://dx.doi.org/10.1136/bjophthalmol-2020-316304]

[21]   Dixon BE, Wools-Kaloustian KK, Fadel WF, *et al.* Symptoms and symptom clusters associated with SARS-CoV-2 infection in community-based populations: Results from a statewide epidemiological study. PLoS One 2021; 16(3): e0241875.

[http://dx.doi.org/10.1371/journal.pone.0241875] [PMID: 33760821]

[22]   Whitaker M, Elliott J, Chadeau-Hyam M, *et al.* Persistent symptoms following SARS-CoV-2 infection in a random community sample of 508,707 people. Medrxiv 2021.
[http://dx.doi.org/10.1101/2021.06.28.21259452]

[23]   Ahamad MM, Aktar S, Rashed-Al-Mahfuz M, *et al.* A machine learning model to identify early stage symptoms of SARS-Cov-2 infected patients. Expert Syst Appl 2020; 160: 113661.
[http://dx.doi.org/10.1016/j.eswa.2020.113661] [PMID: 32834556]

[24]   Chung E, Chow EJ, Wilcox NC, *et al.* Comparison of symptoms and RNA levels in children and adults with SARS-CoV-2 infection in the community setting. JAMA Pediatr 2021; 175(10): e212025.
[http://dx.doi.org/10.1001/jamapediatrics.2021.2025] [PMID: 34115094]

[25]   Available from: https://www.who.int/emergencies/diseases/novel-coronavirus-2019/origins-of-the-virus accessed on 18 January, 2024.

[26]   Singh D, Yi SV. On the origin and evolution of SARS-CoV-2. Exp Mol Med 2021; 53(4): 537-47.
[http://dx.doi.org/10.1038/s12276-021-00604-z] [PMID: 33864026]

[27]   Alwine JC, Casadevall A, Enquist LW, Goodrum FD, Imperiale MJ. A critical analysis of the evidence for the SARS-CoV-2 origin hypotheses. J Virol 2023; 97(4): e00365-23.
[http://dx.doi.org/10.1128/jvi.00365-23] [PMID: 36897089]

[28]   Shaikh SS, Jose AP, Nerkar DA, Vijaykumar KV M, Shaikh SK. COVID-19 pandemic crisis—a complete outline of SARS-CoV-2. Future Journal of Pharmaceutical Sciences 2020; 6(1): 116.
[http://dx.doi.org/10.1186/s43094-020-00133-y] [PMID: 33224993]

[29]   Yao X, Ye F, Zhang M, *et al. In vitro* antiviral activity and projection of optimized dosing design of hydroxychloroquine for the treatment of severe acute respiratory syndrome coronavirus 2 (SARS-CoV-2). Clin Infect Dis 2020; 71(15): 732-9.
[http://dx.doi.org/10.1093/cid/ciaa237] [PMID: 32150618]

[30]   Gasmi A, Peana M, Noor S, *et al.* Chloroquine and hydroxychloroquine in the treatment of COVID-19: the never-ending story. Appl Microbiol Biotechnol 2021; 105(4): 1333-43.
[http://dx.doi.org/10.1007/s00253-021-11094-4] [PMID: 33515285]

[31]   Horby P, Mafham M, Linsell L, *et al.* Effect of hydroxychloroquine in hospitalized patients with Covid-19. N Engl J Med 2020; 383(21): 2030-40.
[http://dx.doi.org/10.1056/NEJMoa2022926] [PMID: 33031652]

[32]   Ledford H. Coronavirus breakthrough: dexamethasone is first drug shown to save lives. Nature 2020; 582(7813): 469.
[http://dx.doi.org/10.1038/d41586-020-01824-5]

[33]   Alunno A, Najm A, Mariette X, *et al.* Immunomodulatory therapies for SARS-CoV-2 infection: a systematic literature review to inform EULAR points to consider. Ann Rheum Dis 2021; 80(6): 803-15.
[http://dx.doi.org/10.1136/annrheumdis-2020-219725] [PMID: 33589438]

[34]   Burrage DR, Koushesh S, Sofat N. Immunomodulatory drugs in the management of SARS-CoV-2. Front Immunol 2020; 11: 1844.
[http://dx.doi.org/10.3389/fimmu.2020.01844] [PMID: 32903555]

[35]   Luo L, Jiang J, Wang C, *et al.* Analysis on herbal medicines utilized for treatment of COVID-19. Acta Pharm Sin B 2020; 10(7): 1192-204.
[http://dx.doi.org/10.1016/j.apsb.2020.05.007] [PMID: 32834949]

[36]   Yang Z, Liu Y, Wang L, *et al.* Traditional Chinese medicine against COVID-19: Role of the gut microbiota. Biomed Pharmacother 2022; 149: 112787.
[http://dx.doi.org/10.1016/j.biopha.2022.112787] [PMID: 35279010]

[37]   Kang X, Jin D, Jiang L, *et al.* Efficacy and mechanisms of traditional Chinese medicine for COVID-

19: a systematic review. Chin Med 2022; 17(1): 30.
[http://dx.doi.org/10.1186/s13020-022-00587-7] [PMID: 35227280]

[38]   Lu S. Timely development of vaccines against SARS-CoV-2. Emerg Microbes Infect 2020; 9(1): 542-4.
[http://dx.doi.org/10.1080/22221751.2020.1737580] [PMID: 32148172]

[39]   Callaway E. The race for coronavirus vaccines: a graphical guide. Nature 2020; 580(7805): 576-7.
[http://dx.doi.org/10.1038/d41586-020-01221-y] [PMID: 32346146]

[40]   Tian X, Li C, Huang A, *et al.* Potent binding of 2019 novel coronavirus spike protein by a SARS coronavirus-specific human monoclonal antibody. Emerg Microbes Infect 2020; 9(1): 382-5.
[http://dx.doi.org/10.1080/22221751.2020.1729069] [PMID: 32065055]

[41]   Kong T, Park JM, Jang JH, *et al.* Immunomodulatory effect of CD200-positive human placenta-derived stem cells in the early phase of stroke. Exp Mol Med 2018; 50(1): e425.
[http://dx.doi.org/10.1038/emm.2017.233] [PMID: 29328072]

[42]   Available from: https://www.who.int/emergencies/diseases/novel-coronavirus-2019/situation-reports accessed on 18 January, 2024.

[43]   Available from: https://www.who.int/emergencies/diseases/novel-coronavirus-2019 accessed on 18 January, 2024.

[44]   Available from: https://www.who.int/docs/default-source/coronaviruse/situation-reports/202001-1-sitrep-1-2019-ncov.pdf?sfvrsn=20a99c10_4 accessed on 18 January, 2024.

[45]   Weekly epidemiological update on COVID-19 - 14 December 2022 (who.int) accessed on 18 January, 2024.

[46]   Yu Kaku, Kaho Okumura, Miguel Padilla-Blanco, Yusuke Kosugi, Keiya Uriu, Alfredo A Hinay Jr., Luo Chen, Arnon Plianchaisuk, Kouji Kobiyama, View ORCID ProfileKen J Ishii, The Genotype to Phenotype Japan (G2P-Japan) Consortium, Jiri Zahradnik, Jumpei Ito, Kei Sato.

[47]   JN. 1 Covid variant: WHO charts its rapid global spread - BBC News accessed on 18 January, 2024.

[48]   Available from: https://www.who.int/emergencies/diseases/novel-coronavirus-2019/advice-for-public?adgroupsurvey={adgroupsurvey}&gclid=Cj0KCQiAkeSsBhDUARIsAK3tief8ISo02JjBbMyCbFnyXGB3A277xQaQbF8pbvkWQmfHEffylIy4JwYaAuXOEALw_wcB accessed on 18 January, 2024.

[49]   Available from: https://www.who.int/emergencies/diseases/novel-coronavirus-2019/covid-19-vaccines/advice accessed on 18 January, 2024.

[50]   Available from: https://www.cdc.gov/coronavirus/2019-ncov/prevent-getting-sick/prevention.html accessed on 18 January, 2024.

CHAPTER 3

Influenza Outbreaks: Predicting Strains, Protecting Yourself, and WHO Guidelines

Simranjeet Kaur[1]**, Akshita Arora**[1]**, Dilpreet Singh**[2]**, Nitin Sharma**[3] **and Amandeep Singh**[1,*]

[1] *Department of Pharmaceutics, ISF College of Pharmacy, Moga, Punjab-142001, India*

[2] *University Institute of Pharma Sciences, Chandigarh University, Gharuan-140413, India*

[3] *Department of Pharmaceutics, Amity Institute of Pharmacy, Amity University, Noida-201301, India*

Abstract: Influenza represents a significant global viral threat, infecting millions annually and leading to hundreds of thousands of deaths. Intermittent influenza pandemics carry substantial risks of illness and death. Belonging to the Orthomyxoviridae family, the influenza virus possesses a segmented, negative-strand RNA genome. The widespread presence of influenza in avian and mammalian species, combined with its segmented genome, creates ongoing possibilities for reassortment events that may result in cross-species transmission. Yearly seasonal influenza outbreaks occur in temperate regions, typically causing common respiratory symptoms like cough, fever, muscle aches, and headache. Pneumonia stands out as the most frequent severe complication, particularly dangerous for young children and older individuals. Antiviral medications are available for influenza treatment and prevention in high-risk groups. While vaccines exist for seasonal influenza prevention, their effectiveness is not ideal. A deeper understanding of early immune responses to influenza is likely to aid in the development of improved influenza vaccines offering broad and lasting immunity.

Keywords: Influenza, Lifecycle, Outbreak, Vaccination, WHO recommendation.

INTRODUCTION

The influenza virus is a part of the *Orthomyxoviridae* family, which acts as major contributor to severe respiratory illness worldwide. It targets vertebrates through four diverse influenza viruses A, B, C, and D [1]. These viruses possess an outer envelope and carry a genome composed of single-strand RNA with a negative polarity and they contribute substantially to the annual mortality rate [2]. Interes-

* **Corresponding author Amandeep Singh:** Department of Pharmaceutics, ISF College of Pharmacy, Moga, Punjab-142001, India; E-mail: ad4singh@gmail.com

tingly, influenza A and B viruses under an electron microscope appear almost identical making them difficult to distinguish. However, the genera can be distinguished by variations in their nucleoprotein antigens and matrix protein [3]. Influenza A virus is extremely pathogenic among the four types of viruses and is capable of infecting a wide range of humans as well as animals and various bird species [4]. In comparison with the other influenza virus types, A type of influenza virus mutates rapidly and also shows greater variability in its antigenicity and virulence [5]. The A type of influenza viruses are further categorized into subtypes depending upon the glycoprotein present on the outermost layer *i.e.,* hemagglutinin (HA) and neuraminidase (NA). These subtypes, such as H1N1 and H3N2, significantly influence the transmission, and pathogenicity of viruses, as well as their ability to evade immune responses [6]. On the other hand, influenza B viruses majorly infect humans, though not as much as influenza A viruses. Influenza C viruses, although less prevalent and typically causing milder symptoms, still cause respiratory infections in humans, particularly in children [7]. Influenza D viruses, a most recent inclusion in the influenza virus categorization, mainly impact cattle and other livestocks. Despite receiving less attention in research compared to other strains, influenza D viruses highlight the zoonotic potential associated with the influenza viruses [8]. The influenza virus is well-known for its capacity to trigger regular seasonal outbreaks and intermittent pandemics, driven by its rapid evolution through processes known as antigenic drift and shift. Antigenic drift encompasses gradual mutations in the virus proteins, resulting in alterations in the strains circulating. Conversely, antigenic shift occurs when entire genome segments, notably those encoding HA genes, are exchanged between different influenza A viruses, giving rise to new subtypes with advantageous characteristics [9]. Influenza viruses are mainly transmitted through airborne droplets produced during coughing or sneezing, and *via* close contact with infected surfaces. Upon infection, these viruses target the respiratory tract, resulting in symptoms such as fever, chills, muscle aches, coughing, and fatigue. In more serious instances, influenza can lead to complications like pneumonia and acute respiratory distress syndrome [10]. Comprehending the characteristics of influenza viruses is essential for crafting successful prevention and management plans. Vaccination is pivotal for mitigating the effects of influenza by conferring immunity against particular strains. This chapter emphasizes the structural components, life cycle, pathophysiology of the influenza virus, and the treatments that are available for their management.

Prevalence

Over time, there has been a consistent increase in cases of influenza virus sequences, with a notable increase throughout the pandemic in 2009 followed by a decrease over the COVID-19 outbreak in 2020 and 2021. Among the genetic sequences of influenza A virus, the H3N2 subtype was dominant for 27 of 34 years, while the H1N1type of influenza dominated in the remaining 7 years [11]. It is important to note that sampling bias in time series data may lead to inaccuracies in describing trends over time. For instance, the drop in cases during the pandemic (COVID-19) constraints may impair sample collection. Factors that may impact sampling biases such as the temporal distribution of data and sample size should be closely monitored [12]. It was observed that H3N2 and H1N1 both are the dominant types of influenza A virus globally, with distinct subtypes distributed across different countries. For example, H9N2, prevalent in China, is mainly found in Asia (90.29%), with smaller proportions in Africa, North America, and Europe [13]. Moreover, the distribution of influenza subtypes varies significantly among different nations, likely influenced by factors like geography, climate, and population mobility. Within the same country, substantial variations in influenza lineage proportions exist among different hosts, possibly related to host species, environmental circumstances, and lifestyle [14]. Both H1N1 and H3N2 subtypes are broadly spread when looking at the top three nations with the largest number of sequences: the United States, China, and the United Kingdom [15].

Structure

Influenza viruses are spherical, pleomorphic particles and filamentous forms can also occur with a diameter of approximately 100 nm. The influenza viruses become inactive on exposure to extreme heat, pH, dryness, and detergents and their viral particles are less stable in their surroundings. The viral particles are enveloped by a lipid bilayer that originates from the host cell. Several glycosylated proteins that emerge from the virus's surface are lodged in the envelope. These three proteins are matrix protein (M), neuraminidase (NA), and hemagglutinin (HA) [16]. The internal structure of influenza A virus is observed in electron micrographs and it is observed that the virus has distinct spikes, which ranges in length from 10 to 14. The HA and NA are present in the ratio 4:1. A helical superstructure, comprising the ribonucleoprotein (RNP) complex, appears beneath the matrix protein (M1), which is located just below the envelope [17]. The nucleoprotein (NP)coated viral RNA segments are linked to the heterotrimeric polymerase complex (PB1, PB2, and PA) to form the RNP complex shown in Fig. (**1**). The virus comprises approximately 1-5% of RNA, 5-8% of them are carbohydrates, 20% are lipids and 70% are proteins [18].

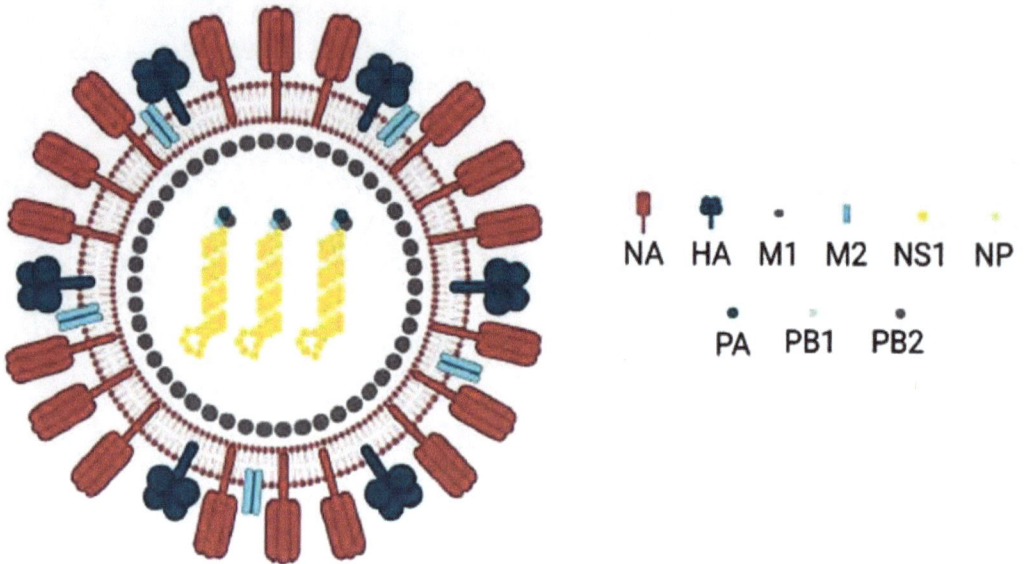

Fig. (1). Structure of influenza virus.

Both A and B influenza viruses have eight different segments containing eight different negative sense, RNA with one strand while influenza C includes seven segments that are termed as viral RNAs, and exist in the form of a structure termed as viral ribonucleoprotein (vRNP) complex. These complexes consist of the RNA strand that further comprises virus's genetic material which is enclosed by NP and adopts a helical configuration, which additionally manages the transcription and replication functions [19]. The viral gene segment contains noncoding regions at both ends. Moreover, these ends act as viral promoters, resulting in replication and transcription [20]. The genomes of the influenza virus are responsible for encoding viral proteins. While the genome primarily codes for 10 major proteins, additional protein variants have been identified from various genome segments [21]. Several RNA molecules are transcribed into messenger RNAs (mRNAs), subsequently split into two chains, each encoding an additional gene product. The comprehensive expression potential of the genome is additionally complex by small viral noncoding RNAs, the functions of which in productive infections remain largely mysterious. The RNA segments, predominantly the largest three, individually carry the genetic code for one of the viral polymerase subunits: PB2, PB1, and PA [22].

Electron microscopy investigations have revealed that the influenza viral RNA polymerase forms a compact structure comprising three genetic products, with PB1 at its core. Among the polymerase subunits, PB1 shows the most conservation, possessing the enzymatic motifs essential for the polymerization activity of RNA [23]. Additionally, within the second segment, an alternate open reading frame generates a supplementary protein called PB1-F2. Exclusive to influenza A, PB1-F2 localizes to mitochondria and demonstrates a pro-apoptotic effect. The PB2 subunit is responsible for recognizing and binding to host mRNA cap structures produced by the cellular transcription machinery, while the acidic protein PA exhibits endonucleolytic activity essential for the viral cap-snatching process [24]. Segment 4 of the influenza virus is responsible for the production of HA proteins, which are trimeric type I integral membrane glycoproteins and prominently present in virions envelop and on infected cell surfaces, serving as a primary target for neutralizing antibodies [25]. Modifications occurring after translation of the HA protein in influenza includes disulphide bond formation, glycosylation, palmitoylation, proteolytic cleavage, and conformational changes. Host cell proteases facilitate the conversion of HAO molecule into its two subunits *i.e.*, HA1 and HA2, and this conversion plays a crucial role in the fusion of HA. Additionally, HA plays a key role in binding virions to the receptor surface of the host cell [26].

Segment 5 of the RNA influenza virus contains genetic instructions for a highly alkaline protein that primarily serves to encapsulate the viral RNA and that protein is known as RNA-binding protein. Additionally, the RNA-binding protein is essential for transporting viral ribonucleoproteins (RNPs) into the nucleus since these RNPs are too large to pass through nuclear pores by passive diffusion [27]. In the later phases of infection, the RNA-binding protein (NP) also interacts with the cytoskeleton and has been observed to attach to filamentous actin [28]. Segment 6 of the influenza virus contains the genetic information for the NA protein [29] and the 7th segment contains information regarding the two proteins *i.e.*, M1 and M2 protein. The M1 protein is produced from a collinear transcript and is crucial for the process of viral budding. Whereas the M2 protein is derived from mRNA and it shows their activity during the entry of the virus [30].

Life Cycle

The lipid bilayer of the influenza virus predominantly comprises three various types of transmembrane proteins hemagglutinin (HA), neuraminidase (NA), and matrix proteins (M). HA contains two different subunits *i.e.*, HA1 and HA2, predominant proteins located on the viral surface [31]. The HA1-mediated receptor serves a vital function in the entry of the influenza virus into the host body as it binds with the sialic acid andafterward undergoes endocytosis that results in the virus uptake. As the endosome matures, the acidic environment of the surrounding results in some conformational changes in HA2, and additionally, the unveiling of the hydrophobic fusion peptide leads to the merging of the endosomal membrane allowing the release of genetic material into the cytoplasm

[32]. Afterward, the vRNPs migrate to the nucleus, where the transcription of vRNA messenger RNA takes place, after which the viral mRNAs are transported into the cytoplasm for translation into various viral proteins [33, 34]. The recently generated nucleoprotein. By the utilization of a complementary RNA (cRNA) intermediate, the newly formed nucleoprotein and RNA-dependent RNA polymerase component were transferred to the nucleus to commence viral RNA replication [35]. These recently copied vRNA molecules can serve for transcription, and replication and are exported from the nucleus. The exportation is facilitated by the chromosome region maintenance 1 (CRM1)-dependent pathway through nuclear pores, with the involvement of viral M1 and nuclear export protein (NEP). Subsequently, progeny virions cluster in the cytoplasm and emerge at the host cell's plasma membrane by budding. Finally, the viral neuraminidase (NA) present on the plasma membrane will remove the sialic acid (SA) residue from glycoproteins and glycolipids, enabling the mature virions to be released from the host cells [36] as shown in Fig. (**2**).

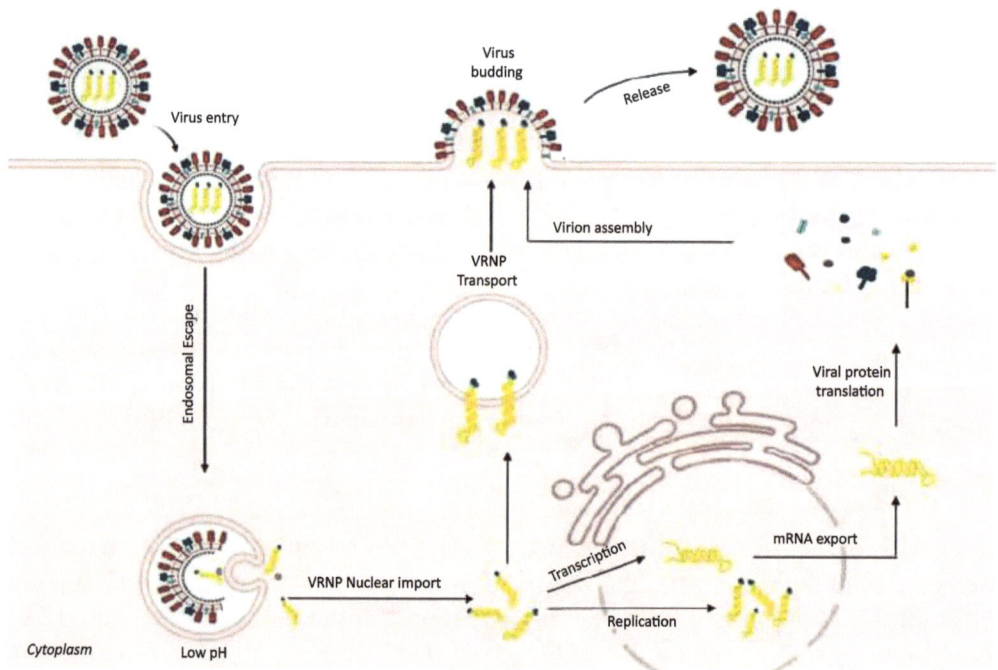

Fig. (2). Lifecycle of influenza virus.

Pathogenesis

The influenza virus is typically transferred via the respiratory pathway while the avian influenza virus is primarily transmitted among birds *via* close contact with faeces through oral and respiratory routes [37]. Viruses primarily reproduce within the epithelial cells that line either the respiratory or intestinal tract. Replication of the virus reached its highest point approximately 48 hours after inoculation and gradually decreased afterward, with minimum shedding occurring over 6-8 days [38]. Mild cases of influenza usually affect the upper respiratory tract and trachea, while severe illness in humans is linked to viral activity in the lower respiratory tract. The influenza virus induces cell apoptosis in epithelial cells *via* different mechanisms. Moreover, epithelial cells that are infected with a virus, release signaling molecules like cytokines and chemokines to attract immune cells such as neutrophils and macrophages, as well as activate neighboring endothelial cells and these cells further produce inflammatory cytokines to a higher extent, which promotes infiltration, damage to the epithelial-endothelial barrier, and subsequent epithelial cell death [39]. Hence, the development of severe influenza results from not only the direct damage caused by the virus itself but also from heightened inflammatory reactions from the host. Consequently, effective treatments should target both viral replication and the inflammatory response within the airways [40].

Prevention and Treatment

Influenza immunization stands as a highly effective therapy to prevent infection. The level of protection for individuals and communities against influenza hinges on the extent of vaccine coverage and uptake, as well as the interplay between the strain antigen present in the vaccine and the circulating strains of influenza [41]. Some research indicates that the influenza vaccine offers up to 60% effectiveness against infection from both Type A and Type B viruses [42]. Basically, there are three types of influenza vaccinations available: influenza vaccine (IIV), live attenuated influenza vaccine (LAIV), and recombinant influenza vaccine. Most of the trivalent vaccines for the 2019-2020 period include components from two types of Influenza A strains and one type of Influenza B [43]. The vaccination of influenza is considered safe for individuals of 6 months and older. The non-adjuvant and adjuvant trivalent influenza vaccine both are recommended for use in individuals over 65 years old [44]. The quadrivalent vaccines for influenza without adjuvant are authorized for individuals aged 6 months and older [45]. A recombinant quadrivalent influenza vaccination is recommended for people over 18 years of age [46]. A quadrivalent live attenuated influenza vaccine (LAIV4) is suitable for healthy individuals aged 2-49 years old, with reported effectiveness in 90% of children unless specifically contraindicated. However, caution is advised as this vaccine is not recommended for use during pregnancy or in individuals with immunodeficiency [47].

Antivirals

Currently, all the guidelines suggest the administration of antiviral medication, particularly in individuals susceptible to serious medical complications. Three primary categories of antiviral medications have been authorized in numerous countries for managing influenza A infections. These include M2 blockers, neuraminidase inhibitors, and polymerase acid inhibitors, all of which hinder viral replication. Moreover, researchers are currently exploring a novel category of drugs known as cap-dependent endonuclease inhibitors [48]. The ongoing research for the development of new antiviral drugs is driven by the rapid evolution of the influenza virus, leading to reduced vaccine effectiveness and the emergence of drug-resistant strains. Research is currently focused on various approaches, including synthetic, biological (bacterial), and plant-derived substances, such as Zanamivir and Oseltamivir [49, 50].

Corticosteroid

Primarily, corticosteroids were given without specific indication to mitigate the inflammatory response in influenza-infected patients. However, subsequent research highlighted their association with higher mortality rates, especially when used at the outset, and an increased risk of hospital-acquired infections. Recently, a phase 3 clinical trial, employing a randomized, double-blind, multicenter design, explored the impact of intravenous hydrocortisone (administered 200 mg dose daily for either 4 or 8 days based on clinical progress) in 800 intensive care unit admitted patients with serious pneumonia [51]. By the 28th day, individuals treated with hydrocortisone exhibited a reduced likelihood of mortality in contrast to those who were given a placebo. Nonetheless, investigations conducted on influenza patients and a recent meta-analysis comprising 10 trials and 6548 individuals with severe influenza pneumonia revealed that corticosteroid treatment was linked to elevated mortality rates, prolonged ICU stays, and heightened occurrence of secondary infections [52]. Hence, using systemic corticosteroids is not advisable for treating ICU patients with influenza pneumonia, backed by limited supporting evidence, underscoring the necessity for further clinical trials. Some researchers propose administering low-dose corticosteroids in cases of septic shock, albeit its occurrence is rare in adequately resuscitated patients. According to expert guidelines, corticosteroids might be considered for patients with ARDS following antiviral treatment and a negative PCR test [53, 54]. Alternative treatments aimed at regulating the inflammatory response, such as statins, n-acetylcysteine, macrolide antibiotics, and cyclooxygenase-2 inhibitors, have shown inefficacy [55].

Monoclonal Antibodies

The development of resistance to existing antiviral medications underscores the urgency of creating novel treatments. Experimental use of monoclonal antibodies (mAb) has shown associations with improved survival rates, reduction in histological alterations, and less severe lung inflammation. Numerous mAbs are presently undergoing different phases of clinical trials and show potential as valuable new resources against the swiftly mutating influenza virus in the foreseeable future [56]. The mAbs are synthesized in labs and exhibit high efficacy towards the specific target antigen or epitope of the antigen. Due to the advancements in molecular biology, structural biology, and bioinformatics, mAbs have evolved significantly, becoming integral elements of immunotherapeutics [57]. Over the past decade, numerous human studies have demonstrated the ability of monoclonal antibodies to effectively bind to and neutralize various strains of influenza A and B viruses. The majority of these antibodies target hemagglutinin, with some currently undergoing assessment in clinical trials. Crucially, findings from these clinical trials suggest that this method is safe and capable of alleviating symptoms associated with influenza [58]. Researchers advised that therapy should commence over the phase of viral replication at its peak level [59]. Almost less than 1% of a biological agent reaches the lung lumen, where the antibodies show their activity by neutralizing the virus and also remove the infected cells with the assistance of immune cells like macrophages, and natural killer cells [60]. The administration of anti-influenza antibodies directly into the lungs could potentially decrease the necessary dosage, potentially resulting in more significant clinical advantages. Additionally, the use of mAb clinically is quite expensive. Therefore, efforts are underway to create more economical approaches for both producing and administering antibodies. The mAbs that are derived from plant source are cost-effective and evaluated through clinical trials [61]. Recent research is exploring innovative techniques for producing and delivering monoclonal antibodies (mAb). This includes methods like introducing nucleotide sequences encoding mAb into the human body through DNA/RNA-based gene therapy or *via* adeno-associated viruses [62, 63].

Antibiotics

A literature study indicates significant variations in the frequency of bacterial co-infections, partly due to differences in the studies and populations examined. The incidence of bacterial co-infection is higher in influenza pneumonia patients with H1N1vIPN. Hence, it is recommended to start empiric antibiotic therapy in such situations while also collecting high-quality respiratory specimens for microbiological examination. It enables the quick termination of antibiotic therapy if microbiological tests come back negative. Reported rates of bacterial co-infection in influenza patients range widely from 2% to 65% across various studies [64]. Biomarkers like procalcitonin (PCT) are valuable for ruling out bacterial co-infection, especially in non-shock patients, and can help guide decisions on discontinuing antibiotic therapy [65]. Streptococcus pneumoniae and Staphylococcus aureus are commonly found bacteria, which justifies the use of initial antibiotic treatment to target these microorganisms. Ceftaroline presents as a viable choice for combating both pneumococcal and staphylococcal infections, even those that are methicillin-resistant [66].

Advanced Treatment Approaches

The shift towards newer targeted strategies has been marked by an emphasis on precision and individualized treatment modalities, stepping beyond traditional drug treatments. One of the forefront approaches includes the use of RNA interference (RNAi) technology, which targets the genetic material of the influenza virus directly, silencing key genes necessary for the virus's replication and spread. This method offers a highly specific way to combat different strains of influenza, potentially reducing the risk of resistance development [67]. Another innovative strategy is the application of CRISPR-Cas9 gene-editing technology to either disrupt viral DNA within infected cells or enhance host cells' resistance to infection. By targeting the influenza virus's genetic makeup, CRISPR-Cas9 can provide a powerful tool for both treatment and prevention, offering hope for a long-term solution against flu outbreaks. Advancements in immunotherapy have also paved the way for new influenza treatments [68]. This involves using engineered antibodies or immune system components to target specific viral antigens, boosting the body's natural defense mechanisms against the virus. Such therapies can offer both therapeutic and prophylactic benefits, especially for high-risk groups and in settings where traditional vaccines are less effective. Vaccine development strategies have also evolved, with a focus on creating universal vaccines that target the more conserved parts of the virus, aiming to provide protection against a broader range of influenza strains over multiple seasons [69]. This approach seeks to mitigate the limitations of current flu vaccines, which must be updated annually to match circulating strains. The World Health Organization (WHO) supports these innovative strategies through its Global Influenza Surveillance and Response System (GISRS), which monitors flu viruses worldwide, providing critical information that informs the development of targeted therapies and vaccines. These newer targeted strategies represent a significant shift in the fight against influenza, offering more effective, long-lasting, and precise options for prevention and treatment, aligning with the WHO's goals for global health security and influenza pandemic preparedness [70].

WHO Recommendation

The World Health Organization (WHO) plays a crucial role in providing recommendations and guidance related to influenza viruses. Some of the key roles of WHO in this regard include the following points.

Surveillance and Monitoring

Effective influenza surveillance and monitoring are crucial for the control of seasonal influenza epidemics and the reduction of the potential effects of influenza pandemics. They also enable early identification, prompt action, and data-driven decision-making. The World Health Organization (WHO) works with laboratories and national health authorities worldwide to track the evolution and transmission of influenza viruses [71].

Preventive Measures

It is perhaps possible to stop the spread of viruses by maintaining good hygiene, which includes washing hands thoroughly with soap, covering the mouth and nose while coughing or sneezing, and refraining from touching the face, eyes, nose, or mouth with unclean hands [72].

Antiviral Treatment

The use of antiviral medicines for the treatment and prevention of influenza, particularly during outbreaks and pandemics ensures effective influenza control and management [73].

Global Coordination

WHO coordinates with various international organizations, to ensure a coordinated global response to influenza outbreaks and pandemics. Some of these organizations are the Centers for Disease Control and Prevention (CDC) in the United States and the European Centre for Disease Prevention and Control (ECDC) in Europe, to ensure a coordinated global response to influenza outbreaks and pandemics [74].

CONCLUSION

Influenza is a highly infectious respiratory illness and it is possible to prevent influenza. It can result in significant problems and fatalities in otherwise healthy people of any age. Differentiating influenza from other respiratory infections presents challenges, particularly in terms of assessing the efficacy of antiviral treatments, leading to delays in their administration. While the influenza vaccination is still the most efficient approach for preventing the infection and its complications, additional, more potent interventions are required for older individuals, who experience the highest incidence of influenza and have lower vaccine effectiveness against severe outcomes.

REFERENCES

[1] Nuwarda RF, Alharbi AA, Kayser V. An overview of influenza viruses and vaccines. Vaccines (Basel) 2021; 9(9): 1032.
[http://dx.doi.org/10.3390/vaccines9091032] [PMID: 34579269]

[2] Krejcova L, Michalek P, Hynek D, Adam V, Kizek R. Structure of influenza viruses, connected with influenza life cycle. J Metallomics Nanotechnol 2015; 2(1): 13-9.

[3] Kumar B, Asha K, Khanna M, Ronsard L, Meseko CA, Sanicas M. The emerging influenza virus threat: status and new prospects for its therapy and control. Arch Virol 2018; 163(4): 831-44.
[http://dx.doi.org/10.1007/s00705-018-3708-y] [PMID: 29322273]

[4] Han AX, de Jong SPJ, Russell CA. Co-evolution of immunity and seasonal influenza viruses. Nat Rev Microbiol 2023; 21(12): 805-17.
[http://dx.doi.org/10.1038/s41579-023-00945-8] [PMID: 37532870]

[5] Sreenivasan CC, Liu R, Gao R, *et al.* Influenza C and D viruses demonstrated a differential respiratory tissue tropism in a comparative pathogenesis study in guinea pigs. J Virol 2023; 97(6): e00356-23.
[http://dx.doi.org/10.1128/jvi.00356-23] [PMID: 37199648]

[6] Kackos CM, DeBeauchamp J, Davitt CJ, Lonzaric J, Sealy RE, Hurwitz JL. Seasonal quadrivalent mRNA vaccine prevents and mitigates influenza infection. npj. Vaccines (Basel) 2023; 8(1): 157.
[PMID: 36680002]

[7] Peteranderl C, Herold S, Schmoldt C, Eds. Human influenza virus infections Seminars in respiratory and critical care medicine. Thieme Medical Publishers 2016.

[8] Liu R, Sheng Z, Huang C, Wang D, Li F. Influenza D virus. Curr Opin Virol 2020; 44: 154-61.
[http://dx.doi.org/10.1016/j.coviro.2020.08.004] [PMID: 32932215]

[9] Shao W, Li X, Goraya M, Wang S, Chen JL. Evolution of influenza a virus by mutation and re-assortment. Int J Mol Sci 2017; 18(8): 1650.
[http://dx.doi.org/10.3390/ijms18081650] [PMID: 28783091]

[10] Mehta D, Spearman P. Influenza viruses molecular medical microbiology. Elsevier 2024; pp. 2357-73.
[http://dx.doi.org/10.1016/B978-0-12-818619-0.00148-9]

[11] Zachreson C, Fair KM, Cliff OM, Harding N, Piraveenan M, Prokopenko M. Urbanization affects peak timing, prevalence, and bimodality of influenza pandemics in Australia: Results of a census-calibrated model. Sci Adv 2018; 4(12): eaau5294.
[http://dx.doi.org/10.1126/sciadv.aau5294] [PMID: 30547086]

[12] Gass JD Jr, Dusek RJ, Hall JS, *et al.* Global dissemination of influenza A virus is driven by wild bird migration through arctic and subarctic zones. Mol Ecol 2023; 32(1): 198-213.
[http://dx.doi.org/10.1111/mec.16738] [PMID: 36239465]

[13] Dhanasekaran V, Sullivan S, Edwards KM, *et al.* Human seasonal influenza under COVID-19 and the potential consequences of influenza lineage elimination. Nat Commun 2022; 13(1): 1721.
[http://dx.doi.org/10.1038/s41467-022-29402-5] [PMID: 35361789]

[14] Lam TTY, Zhou B, Wang J, *et al.* Dissemination, divergence and establishment of H7N9 influenza viruses in China. Nature 2015; 522(7554): 102-5.
[http://dx.doi.org/10.1038/nature14348] [PMID: 25762140]

[15] Rejmanek D, Hosseini PR, Mazet JAK, Daszak P, Goldstein T. Evolutionary dynamics and global

diversity of influenza A virus. J Virol 2015; 89(21): 10993-1001.
[http://dx.doi.org/10.1128/JVI.01573-15] [PMID: 26311890]

[16]   Bhalerao U, Mavi AK, Manglic S. Sakshi, Chowdhury S, Kumar U An updated review on influenza viruses Emerging Human Viral Diseases. Respiratory and Haemorrhagic Fever 2023; Vol. I: pp. 71-106.

[17]   Carter T, Iqbal M. The influenza a virus replication cycle: a comprehensive review. Viruses 2024; 16(2): 316.
[http://dx.doi.org/10.3390/v16020316] [PMID: 38400091]

[18]   Blake ME, Kleinpeter AB, Jureka AS, Petit CM. Structural investigations of interactions between the influenza a virus NS1 and host cellular proteins. Viruses 2023; 15(10): 2063.
[http://dx.doi.org/10.3390/v15102063] [PMID: 37896840]

[19]   Langer D, Mlynarczyk DT, Dlugaszewska J, Tykarska E. Potential of glycyrrhizic and glycyrrhetinic acids against influenza type A and B viruses: A perspective to develop new anti-influenza compounds and drug delivery systems. Eur J Med Chem 2023; 246: 114934.
[http://dx.doi.org/10.1016/j.ejmech.2022.114934] [PMID: 36455358]

[20]   Chauhan RP, Gordon ML. An overview of influenza A virus genes, protein functions, and replication cycle highlighting important updates. Virus Genes 2022; 58(4): 255-69.
[http://dx.doi.org/10.1007/s11262-022-01904-w] [PMID: 35471490]

[21]   Martín-Benito J, Ortín J. Influenza virus transcription and replication Advances in virus research 87. Elsevier 2013; pp. 113-37.

[22]   Reguera D, de Pablo PJ, Abrescia NGA, *et al.* Physical virology in spain. Biophysica 2023; 3(4): 598-619.
[http://dx.doi.org/10.3390/biophysica3040041]

[23]   Griffin EF, Tompkins SM. Fitness determinants of influenza a viruses. Viruses 2023; 15(9): 1959.
[http://dx.doi.org/10.3390/v15091959] [PMID: 37766365]

[24]   Jiang L, Chen H, Li C. Advances in deciphering the interactions between viral proteins of influenza A virus and host cellular proteins. Cell Insight 2023; 2(2): 100079.
[http://dx.doi.org/10.1016/j.cellin.2023.100079] [PMID: 37193064]

[25]   Li D, Lin Q, Luo F, Wang H. Insights into the Structure, Metabolism, Biological Functions and Molecular Mechanisms of Sialic Acid: A Review. Foods 2023; 13(1): 145.
[http://dx.doi.org/10.3390/foods13010145] [PMID: 38201173]

[26]   Liang Y. Pathogenicity and virulence of influenza. Virulence 2023; 14(1): 2223057.
[http://dx.doi.org/10.1080/21505594.2023.2223057] [PMID: 37339323]

[27]   Singh P, Sodhi KK, Bali AK, Shree P. Influenza A virus and its antiviral drug treatment options. Medicine in Microecology 2023; p. 100083.

[28]   Lal SK. Influenza A Virus: Host–Virus Relationships. MDPI 2020; p. 870.

[29]   Husain M. Influenza virus host restriction factors: the ISGs and Non-ISGs. Pathogens 2024; 13(2): 127.
[http://dx.doi.org/10.3390/pathogens13020127] [PMID: 38392865]

[30]   Sun X, Ma H, Wang X, *et al.* Broadly neutralizing antibodies to combat influenza virus infection. Antiviral Res 2024; 221: 105785.
[http://dx.doi.org/10.1016/j.antiviral.2023.105785] [PMID: 38145757]

[31]   Chen Z, Cui Q, Caffrey M, Rong L, Du R. Small molecule inhibitors of influenza virus entry. Pharmaceuticals (Basel) 2021; 14(6): 587.
[http://dx.doi.org/10.3390/ph14060587] [PMID: 34207368]

[32]   Luo M. Influenza virus entry. Viral molecular machines. 2012: 201-21.
[http://dx.doi.org/10.1007/978-1-4614-0980-9_9]

[33]   Reich S, Guilligay D, Pflug A, *et al.* Structural insight into cap-snatching and RNA synthesis by influenza polymerase. Nature 2014; 516(7531): 361-6.
[http://dx.doi.org/10.1038/nature14009] [PMID: 25409151]

[34]   Eisfeld AJ, Neumann G, Kawaoka Y. At the centre: influenza A virus ribonucleoproteins. Nat Rev Microbiol 2015; 13(1): 28-41.
[http://dx.doi.org/10.1038/nrmicro3367] [PMID: 25417656]

[35]   Luo W, Zhang J, Liang L, *et al.* Phospholipid scramblase 1 interacts with influenza A virus NP, impairing its nuclear import and thereby suppressing virus replication. PLoS Pathog 2018; 14(1): e1006851.
[http://dx.doi.org/10.1371/journal.ppat.1006851] [PMID: 29352288]

[36]   Chaimayo C, Hayashi T, Underwood A, Hodges E, Takimoto T. Selective incorporation of vRNP into influenza A virions determined by its specific interaction with M1 protein. Virology 2017; 505: 23-32.
[http://dx.doi.org/10.1016/j.virol.2017.02.008] [PMID: 28219018]

[37]   Hutchinson EC. Influenza Virus. Trends Microbiol 2018; 26(9): 809-10.
[http://dx.doi.org/10.1016/j.tim.2018.05.013] [PMID: 29909041]

[38]   Taubenberger JK, Morens DM. The pathology of influenza virus infections. Annu Rev Pathol 2008; 3(1): 499-522.
[http://dx.doi.org/10.1146/annurev.pathmechdis.3.121806.154316] [PMID: 18039138]

[39]   Wei F, Gao C, Wang Y. The role of influenza A virus-induced hypercytokinemia. Crit Rev Microbiol 2022; 48(2): 240-56.
[http://dx.doi.org/10.1080/1040841X.2021.1960482] [PMID: 34353210]

[40]   Flerlage T, Boyd DF, Meliopoulos V, Thomas PG, Schultz-Cherry S. Influenza virus and SARS-Co-2: pathogenesis and host responses in the respiratory tract. Nat Rev Microbiol 2021; 19(7): 425-41.
[http://dx.doi.org/10.1038/s41579-021-00542-7] [PMID: 33824495]

[41]   Paules CI, Fauci AS. Influenza vaccines: good, but we can do better. J Infect Dis 2019; 219 (Suppl. 1): S1-4.
[http://dx.doi.org/10.1093/infdis/jiy633] [PMID: 30715469]

[42]   Lall D, Cason E, Pasquel FJ, Ali MK, Narayan KMV. Effectiveness of influenza vaccination for individuals with chronic obstructive pulmonary disease (COPD) in low-and middle-income countries. COPD 2016; 13(1): 93-9.
[http://dx.doi.org/10.3109/15412555.2015.1043518] [PMID: 26418892]

[43]   Xu XiYan XX, Blanton L, Elal A, Alabi N, Barnes J, Biggerstaff M. Update: influenza activity in the United States during the 2018-19 season and composition of the 2019-20 influenza vaccine. 2019.

[44]   Grohskopf LA, Alyanak E, Broder KR, Walter EB, Fry AM, Jernigan DB. Prevention and control of seasonal influenza with vaccines: recommendations of the Advisory Committee on Immunization Practices—United States, 2019–20 influenza season. MMWR Recomm Rep 2019; 68(3): 1-21.
[http://dx.doi.org/10.15585/mmwr.rr6803a1] [PMID: 31441906]

[45]   Montomoli E, Torelli A, Manini I, Gianchecchi E. Immunogenicity and safety of the new inactivated quadrivalent influenza vaccine vaxigrip tetra: preliminary results in children≥ 6 months and older adults. Vaccines (Basel) 2018; 6(1): 14.
[http://dx.doi.org/10.3390/vaccines6010014] [PMID: 29518013]

[46]   Cruz-Valdez A, Valdez-Zapata G, Patel SS, *et al.* MF59-adjuvanted influenza vaccine (FLUAD®) elicits higher immune responses than a non-adjuvanted influenza vaccine (Fluzone®): A randomized, multicenter, Phase III pediatric trial in Mexico. Hum Vaccin Immunother 2018; 14(2): 386-95.
[http://dx.doi.org/10.1080/21645515.2017.1373227] [PMID: 28925801]

[47]   Strohmeier S, Amanat F, Zhu X, *et al.* A novel recombinant influenza virus neuraminidase vaccine candidate stabilized by a measles virus phosphoprotein tetramerization domain provides robust protection from virus challenge in the mouse model. MBio 2021; 12(6): e02241-21.

[http://dx.doi.org/10.1128/mBio.02241-21] [PMID: 34809451]

[48]   Świerczyńska M, Mirowska-Guzel DM, Pindelska E. Antiviral drugs in influenza. Int J Environ Res Public Health 2022; 19(5): 3018.
       [http://dx.doi.org/10.3390/ijerph19053018] [PMID: 35270708]

[49]   Beigel JH, Bao Y, Beeler J, *et al.* Oseltamivir, amantadine, and ribavirin combination antiviral therapy *versus* oseltamivir monotherapy for the treatment of influenza: a multicentre, double-blind, randomised phase 2 trial. Lancet Infect Dis 2017; 17(12): 1255-65.
       [http://dx.doi.org/10.1016/S1473-3099(17)30476-0] [PMID: 28958678]

[50]   Nakamura S, Miyazaki T, Izumikawa K, Kakeya H, Saisho Y, Yanagihara K, Eds. Efficacy and safety of intravenous peramivir compared with oseltamivir in high-risk patients infected with influenza A and B viruses: a multicenter randomized controlled study Open Forum Infectious Diseases. Oxford University Press US 2017.

[51]   Dequin PF, Meziani F, Quenot JP, *et al.* Hydrocortisone in severe community-acquired pneumonia. N Engl J Med 2023; 388(21): 1931-41.
       [http://dx.doi.org/10.1056/NEJMoa2215145] [PMID: 36942789]

[52]   Ni Y-N, Chen G, Sun J, Liang B-M, Liang Z-A. The effect of corticosteroids on mortality of patients with influenza pneumonia: a systematic review and meta-analysis. Crit Care 2019; 23: 1-9.

[53]   Board GPM. A world at risk. Geneva: World Health Organization and the World Bank. 2019.

[54]   Torres A, Loeches IM, Sligl W, Lee N. Severe flu management: a point of view. Intensive Care Med 2020; 46(2): 153-62.
       [http://dx.doi.org/10.1007/s00134-019-05868-8] [PMID: 31912206]

[55]   Valenzuela-Sánchez F, Valenzuela-Méndez B, Rodríguez-Gutiérrez JF, Rello J. Personalized medicine in severe influenza. Eur J Clin Microbiol Infect Dis 2016; 35(6): 893-7.
       [http://dx.doi.org/10.1007/s10096-016-2611-2] [PMID: 26936615]

[56]   Nosaka N, Yashiro M, Yamada M, *et al.* Anti-high mobility group box-1 monoclonal antibody treatment provides protection against influenza A virus (H1N1)-induced pneumonia in mice. Crit Care 2015; 19(1): 249.
       [http://dx.doi.org/10.1186/s13054-015-0983-9] [PMID: 26067826]

[57]   Gao Y, Huang X, Zhu Y, Lv Z. A brief review of monoclonal antibody technology and its representative applications in immunoassays. J Immunoassay Immunochem 2018; 39(4): 351-64.
       [http://dx.doi.org/10.1080/15321819.2018.1515775] [PMID: 30204067]

[58]   Sedeyn K, Saelens X. New antibody-based prevention and treatment options for influenza. Antiviral Res 2019; 170: 104562.
       [http://dx.doi.org/10.1016/j.antiviral.2019.104562] [PMID: 31323236]

[59]   Beigel JH, Nam HH, Adams PL, *et al.* Advances in respiratory virus therapeutics – A meeting report from the 6th isirv Antiviral Group conference. Antiviral Res 2019; 167: 45-67.
       [http://dx.doi.org/10.1016/j.antiviral.2019.04.006] [PMID: 30974127]

[60]   Hart TK, Cook RM, Zia-Amirhosseini P, *et al.* Preclinical efficacy and safety of mepolizumab (SB-240563), a humanized monoclonal antibody to IL-5, in cynomolgus monkeys. J Allergy Clin Immunol 2001; 108(2): 250-7.
       [http://dx.doi.org/10.1067/mai.2001.116576] [PMID: 11496242]

[61]   Chen Q. Development of plant-made monoclonal antibodies against viral infections. Curr Opin Virol 2022; 52: 148-60.
       [http://dx.doi.org/10.1016/j.coviro.2021.12.005] [PMID: 34933212]

[62]   Sun X, Ling Z, Yang Z, Sun B. Broad neutralizing antibody-based strategies to tackle influenza. Curr Opin Virol 2022; 53: 101207.
       [http://dx.doi.org/10.1016/j.coviro.2022.101207] [PMID: 35131735]

[63] Wang Q, Huang Z. Editorial overview: Anti-viral strategies: Human antibody immune response and antibody-based therapy against viruses. Curr Opin Virol 2022; 55: 101247.
[http://dx.doi.org/10.1016/j.coviro.2022.101247] [PMID: 35803202]

[64] Rynda-Apple A, Robinson KM, Alcorn JF. Influenza and bacterial superinfection: illuminating the immunologic mechanisms of disease. Infect Immun 2015; 83(10): 3764-70.
[http://dx.doi.org/10.1128/IAI.00298-15] [PMID: 26216421]

[65] Rodríguez AH, Avilés-Jurado FX, Díaz E, *et al.* Procalcitonin (PCT) levels for ruling-out bacterial coinfection in ICU patients with influenza: A CHAID decision-tree analysis. J Infect 2016; 72(2): 143-51.
[http://dx.doi.org/10.1016/j.jinf.2015.11.007] [PMID: 26702737]

[66] Klein EY, Monteforte B, Gupta A, *et al.* The frequency of influenza and bacterial coinfection: a systematic review and meta-analysis. Influenza Other Respir Viruses 2016; 10(5): 394-403.
[http://dx.doi.org/10.1111/irv.12398] [PMID: 27232677]

[67] Shi Y, Shi X, Liang J, *et al.* Aggravated MRSA pneumonia secondary to influenza A virus infection is derived from decreased expression of IL-1β. J Med Virol 2020; 92(12): 3047-56.
[http://dx.doi.org/10.1002/jmv.26329] [PMID: 32697385]

[68] Nicholson EG, Munoz FM. A review of therapeutics in clinical development for respiratory syncytial virus and influenza in children. Clin Ther 2018; 40(8): 1268-81.
[http://dx.doi.org/10.1016/j.clinthera.2018.06.014] [PMID: 30077340]

[69] Mady A, Ramadan OS, Yousef A, Mandourah Y, Amr AA, Kherallah M. Clinical experience with severe 2009 H1N1 influenza in the intensive care unit at King Saud Medical City, Saudi Arabia. J Infect Public Health 2012; 5(1): 52-6.
[http://dx.doi.org/10.1016/j.jiph.2011.10.005] [PMID: 22341843]

[70] Hay AJ, McCauley JW. The WHO global influenza surveillance and response system (GISRS)—A future perspective. Influenza Other Respir Viruses 2018; 12(5): 551-7.
[http://dx.doi.org/10.1111/irv.12565] [PMID: 29722140]

[71] Available from: https://www.emro.who.int/health-topics/influenza/influenza-surveillance.html

[72] Available from: https://iris.who.int/bitstream/handle/10665/352453/9789240040816eng.pdf?sequence=1&isAllowed=y

[73] Available from: https://www.who.int/europe/health-topics/influenza-seasonal#tab=tab_2

[74] Available from: https://www.afro.who.int/health-topics/influenza

CHAPTER 4

Combating Dengue: A Look at the Characteristics, Prevalence, Treatment Approaches, and WHO Recommendations

Akshita Arora[1], Simranjeet Kaur[1], Nitin Sharma[2], Dilpreet Singh[3] and **Amandeep Singh[1,*]**

[1] *Department of Pharmaceutics, ISF College of Pharmacy, Moga, Punjab-142001, India*

[2] *Department of Pharmaceutics, Amity Institute of Pharmacy, Amity University, Noida-201301, India*

[3] *University Institute of Pharma Sciences, Chandigarh University, Gharuan-140413, India*

Abstract: The dengue virus, which causes dengue, is a viral illness spread by arthropods and a severe worldwide public health concern. There are four unique serotypes of the dengue virus. Every year, millions of instances are recorded globally, and many result in deaths. The genetic material of the encapsulated dengue virus, which belongs to the Flaviviridae family, is made up of positive-sense single-stranded RNA. The range of symptoms includes low-grade fever as well as more serious illnesses including dengue haemorrhagic fever, thrombocytopenia, and increased vascular permeability. It is vital to undertake urgent laboratory diagnostic testing to confirm the condition. Examples of diagnostic approaches include virus identification in serological testing and RNA amplification using PCR. Dengue cannot presently be treated or avoided with antiviral medicines owing to licensing difficulties. The only dengue virus vaccine that has been approved is now available: dengvaxia. This book chapter aims to provide insights into the structure, pathophysiology, symptoms, major affected organs, mitigation strategies, and treatment approaches for the dengue virus.

Keywords: Aedes aegypti mosquito, Antiviral, Diagnosis, Dengue virus (DENV), Dengue fever, Viral infection process, WHO recommendation.

INTRODUCTION

The Dengue virus (DENV), a mosquito-borne ailment, has affected a significant portion of the global population. Endemic to over 100 nations across tropical and subtropical zones, including regions such as Spain, Portugal, Africa, the southern

* **Corresponding author Amandeep Singh:** Department of Pharmaceutics, ISF College of Pharmacy, Moga, Punjab-142001, India; E-mail: ad4singh@gmail.com

USA, and Europe, dengue poses a widespread threat. As per WHO's recent data, the yearly dengue cases include 100 to 400 million cases, resulting in around 22,000 fatalities. While the majority, comprising 80%, experience mild or no symptoms, 20% endure severe dengue fever, contributing to the aforementioned mortality rate [1]. DENV belongs to the *Flaviviridae* family and encompasses four distinct types (DENV-1,2, 3, and 4) [2]. The following risk factors are believed to be the primary contributors to the disease including genetic changes from zoonotic strains to human strains [3], mutations in DENV [4], and climate changes [5]. Transmission to humans primarily occurs through mosquito bites, predominantly by the species *Aedes aegypti (A. aegypti)*. The signs of DENV include high fever, joint pain, abdominal pain, vomiting, and loss of appetite. However, severe cases can cause plasma leakage, haemorrhage, dengue shock syndrome, thrombocytopenia, mucosal bleeding, and myalgia [6]. Although the DENV poses a significant health threat, there is currently only one FDA-approved vaccine available, Dengvaxia (CYD-TDV), registered in 20 countries. Many potential antiviral drugs have failed to advance to clinical trials due to shortcomings in their physical and pharmacokinetic properties. Among those that have undergone clinical trials, including chloroquine, prednisolone, lovastatin, and celgosivir, none have demonstrated significant reductions in viral infection [7]. This chapter delves into the evolution of the dengue virus, its prevalence, structure, and pathogenesis, along with the exploration of various therapeutic and control strategies aimed at enhancing dengue prevention and control measures.

Prevalence and Outbreaks of Dengue

Over the previous 20 years, dengue cases have climbed rapidly, from 505,430 in 2000 to over 2.4 million in 2010 and 5.2 million in 2019. America, Southeast Asia, and the Western Pacific are currently in danger of going extinct as a consequence of this [8]. As per WHO's latest data, American regions have experienced the highest number of dengue cases ranging from 1.5 million to 16.2 million in the last 40 years [9]. In 2023, America accounted for 565,911 infections, including 7,653 severe cases, and 2,340 fatalities of dengue virus. The regions of the Americas reported 2,811,433 cases of dengue in 2022, compared to 28203 severe cases and 1823 fatalities in 2019. Numerous regions across America, notably Brazil, Argentina, Colombia, Costa Rica, Mexico, Panama, and Peru experienced severe outbreaks in 2023. Brazil recorded the highest incidence of dengue cases, 2376522, followed by Peru with 188326 cases, Bolivia with 133779 cases, and Argentina with 126431 cases. Contrarily, Colombia, Mexico, and Panama reported 50818, 31549, and 3176 cases, respectively [10]. Unlike America, DENV also poses a significant health burden in Southeast Asian regions including Myanmar, Sri Lanka, Thailand, and the Philippines [11]. The recent data shows, an estimated 2.9 million dengue outbreaks and 5906 deaths annually in Southeast Asia [12]. Between 2015 and 2019, dengue cases in the region increased by 46%, rising from 451442 to 658301, while mortality decreased by 2% during the same period [13]. The Philippines reported the highest number of dengue cases 420,000 in 2019, followed by Thailand (129,906 cases), Malaysia (88,074 cases), and Myanmar (4,121 cases). Apart from America and the Southeast Asian regions, concurrent infections have been reported in Western Pacific countries also. The cases were found to be 430023 in 2013 and substantially increased to 479263 cases in 2019. Large-scale outbreaks with significant rises in the number of illnesses were documented in many of the region's nations between 2013 and 2019. In 2019, the country with the most dengue cases (68597) was followed by China (22188 cases).

Structure of Dengue Virus

The genome is a single positive-stranded RNA with a length of 11 kilobases (kb). The DENV is comprised of both structural and non-structural proteins. The capsid (C), envelope (E), and membrane (M) are the structural proteins; NS1, NS2A, NS2B, NS3, NS4A, and NS4B are the non-structural (NS) proteins [14] shown in Fig. (**1**). Protein C is composed of 100 amino acid residues and molecular weight 12 kDa. It contributes to the packaging of the viral genetic material. Protein E is the major viral protein responsible for virus assembly, hemagglutination, neutralization, and receptor binding. It contains 495 amino acid residues rich in hydrophobic residues and glycine and has a molecular weight of 50 kDa. Protein M, a glycosylated protein with a molecular weight of 18.5 kDa, functions to ensure that the E protein is assembled and folded appropriately [15]. Non-structure proteins are involved in various activities such as replication, immunological regulation, and protein cleavage. NS1 protein has a molecular weight of 46 kDa and it is involved in viral RNA replication and induction of humoral immune response [16]. NS2A and NS4A are hydrophobic integral membrane proteins responsible for RNA replication [17, 18]. NS2B is also a hydrophobic protein, which is a co-factor for the NS3 enzyme. NS3 is a multifunctional protein with a molecular weight of 70kDa. It performs the processing of polyproteins and hydrolysis of ATP as an energy source. NS5 is the largest protein with a molecular weight of 105 kDa, which is involved in RNA production [19].

The DENV RNA genome also carries an open reading frame (ORF) that codes for a 3390-residue polyprotein. Two untranslated regions (UTRs) encircle this ORF: the 3'-UTR, which has 114–650 nucleotides, and the 5'-UTR, which has 95–135 nucleotides. RNA interaction, translation, and viral assembly are all dependent on the secondary structures of these UTRs during replication [20]. The 5' terminal of the genome may contain three principal domains: stem-loop A (SLA), short stem-loop B (SLB), and 5'CS. Domain I: The RNA-dependent RNA polymerase (NS5) detects key structures in the SLA sub-regions (S1, S2, and S3), as well as a top loop (TL) and a side stem-loop (SSL), during viral RNA synthesis. Flaviviruses with S3 and the side stem-loop are the most diverse among them. Short stem-loop B (SLB), a 16-nucleotide domain II, terminates at the translation start codon AUG, which bears the CS 5; UAR. When the 5'UAR and 5'CS hybridize with their 3' UTR counterparts, RNA interactions for genome cyclization occur because of the nucleotide makeup of Domain III, the 5' CS. Three distinct structural elements are found at the 3' terminal: the dumbbell (DB), the conserved sequence (CS), and the stem loop (SL). The stop codon is followed by the SL domain. Domain II appears as tandem duplicates and has a distinctive dumbbell form. The conserved CS2 and its repeating CS2 (RCS2) sequences are included in this domain. In a similar fashion, Domain III has a terminal 3'SL structure following a CS1 element. Long-range interactions between RNA molecules are considerably assisted by CS1, notably during the process of genome end cyclization. The length of the 3' terminal varies across different serotypes: specifically, it consists of 470, 450, 430, and 385 nucleotides in DENV1, 2, 3, and 4, respectively [21, 22].

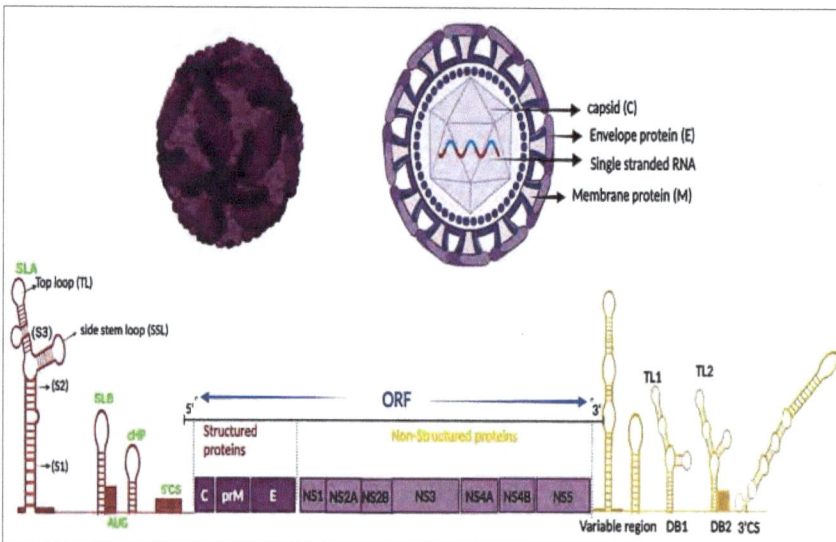

Fig. (1). Structure of dengue virus.

Pathophysiology

The life cycle of DENV embarks as the arthropod stings the individual, as shown in Fig. (**2**). Virions make their way into the human body through various avenues, including fusion, diffusion, micropinocytosis, and endocytosis, facilitated by their interaction with receptors such as DC-SIGN, PS receptors, TIM, Fcγ receptors, and TAM family receptors like TYRO3, AXL, or MERT [23]. Primarily, DENV enters into host cells through receptor-mediated pathways, often utilizing the Fc receptors. The virus remains inside the endosome after it has found its way farther into the host cell. Following internalization, the E protein suffers a conformational change that facilitates membrane fusion due to the acidic environment within the endosome. This stage leads in the release of the viral nucleocapsid into the cytoplasm, where it uncoils and releases the DNA. The viral DNA is subsequently transported to the endoplasmic reticulum (ER) *via* cytoplasmic transport machinery. The ER is the location of translation, where it creates separate structural and non-structural proteins. New positive RNA strands are generated and the genome is enclosed in capsid proteins in the host cell's cytoplasm following viral replication. Subsequently, membrane protein undergoes proteolysis within the Golgi apparatus, which starts off E's rearrangement, homodimerization, and maturation into viral particles. When the fully mature enveloped virus buds off, it is liberated into extracellular spaces and has the capacity to infect surrounding host cells [1, 24].

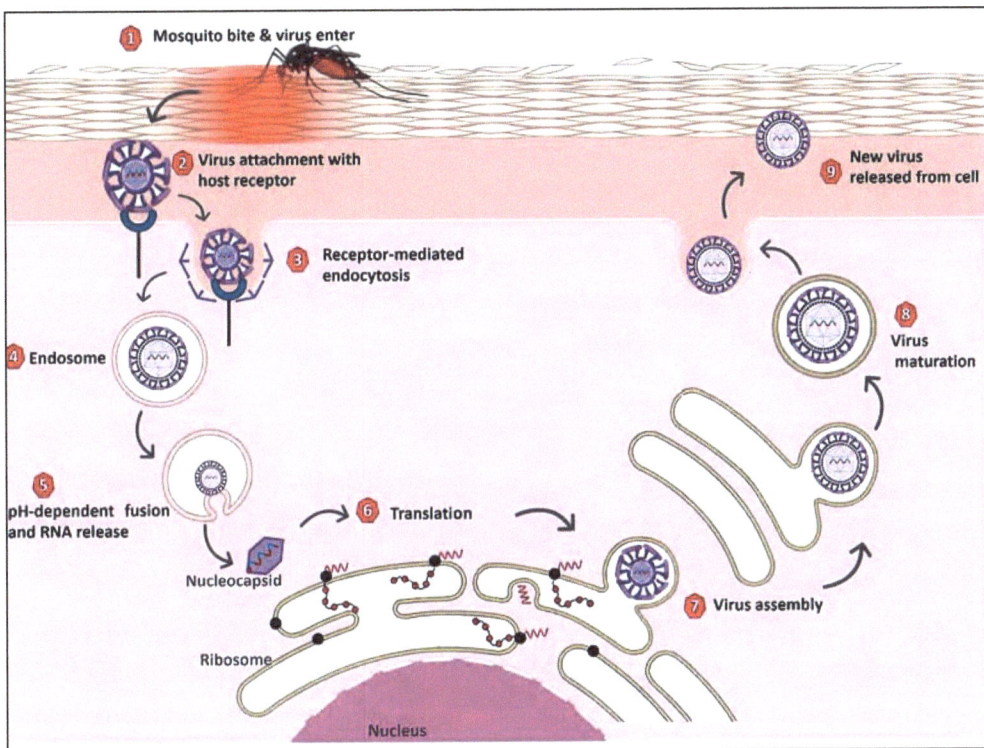

Fig. (2). Life cycle of dengue virus.

Clinical Signs and Symptoms of Dengue

Bite-by-bite transmission of the mosquito-borne flavivirus DENV is predominantly transmitted by Aegypti mosquitoes. The illness is internationally significant, especially in tropical and subtropical locations, where it appears in a broad variety of clinical signs and symptoms that vary in severity. Many persons infected with the dengue virus may initially exhibit little to no symptoms at all, which may be easily mistaken for indications of other illnesses. A high fever, up to 104°F (40°C), is frequently the initial indication of the sickness. Severe headaches, soreness behind the eyes, aches in the muscles and joints, and tiredness are among potential adverse effects. Because these symptoms generate intense agony in the muscles and joints, they are frequently referred to as "breakbone fever". One conspicuous symptom of dengue fever is a measles-like rash that appears two to five days after the fever initially begins. It could expand to the face, arms, and legs from the torso. Additionally, some people may suffer from lymphadenopathy, swollen glands, nausea, or vomiting. Severe dengue, commonly referred to as dengue shock syndrome (DSS) or dengue haemorrhagic fever (DHF), is a rare but severe form of the illness that is marked by organ failure, breathing problems, plasma leakage, fluid buildup, and severe bleeding. Severe dengue fever warning symptoms include extended vomiting, acute

stomach pain, fast breathing, bleeding gums, exhaustion, restlessness, and blood in the faeces or vomit. These severe symptoms are a medical emergency, requiring immediate hospitalization due to the risk of shock and organ failure. The broad spectrum of dengue symptoms emphasizes the need for early detection and treatment to manage the disease effectively and prevent its progression to more severe forms [25-29].

DIAGNOSIS

Virus Isolation

Virus isolation stands as a cornerstone in virological analysis, employing diverse approaches such as introducing specimens (blood, plasma, cerebrospinal fluid, and serum) into mosquitoes or the cerebral tissue of mice, alongside *in vitro* cell line cultures. Among the mammalian cell lines favoured for this purpose are LLCMK2, Vero, and BHK-21 cells, while mosquito cell lines including Tra-284, AP64, C6/36, and CLA-1 cells are commonly utilized [30, 31]. While regarded as the gold standard technique due to its exceptional specificity, virus isolation does present several challenges. These include its time-intensive nature, susceptibility to sample contamination, reliance on sophisticated equipment, intricate procedures, and the necessity for highly skilled personnel. Furthermore, the timing of blood sample collection from infected individuals plays a crucial role, with samples obtained within 5 days of illness onset yielding more favourable outcomes compared to those collected at later stages [32].

Polymerase Chain Reaction (PCR)

PCR, a widely embraced molecular technique, stands as a cornerstone in detecting DENV. In this method, specimens from individuals are collected, and viral RNA is meticulously extracted. Subsequently, this RNA undergoes reverse transcription into complementary DNA (cDNA), followed by amplification utilizing primers targeting conserved regions of the DENV genome. Amplified DNA is then identified through fluorescence-based approaches, with positive results confirming virus' presence [33]. Among the many benefits of this approach are serotype discrimination, high sensitivity, robustness, and repeatability. However, its implementation is hindered due to its high cost, dependence on specialized technology, necessitating highly skilled individuals, and complexity of procedures [34].

Serological Detection

Serological detection methods are commonly employed to distinguish primary and secondary DENV infections contributing to understanding its transmission dynamics. These include a broad variety of tests, such as the enzyme-linked immunosorbent assay (ELISA), Western blotting, dot-blot assays, complement fixation tests, hemagglutination inhibition (HI) assay, and indirect immunofluorescent antibody tests. Among these, ELISA is commonly used to detect anti-DENV IgM and IgG antibodies, notably MAC-ELISA and GAC ELISA. Since IgM forms during the first three to five days of infection, anti-dengue IgM antibodies may be successfully identified during this time. On the other hand, IgG antibodies start to show up in secondary infections 10 to 15 days after the commencement of symptoms [35]. The ratio of IgM to IgG during the acute phase may assist in detecting primary or secondary infection. However, serological detection *via* IgM and IgG assays faces challenges due to cross-reactivity among flaviviruses [36].

TREATMENTS AVAILABLE

Antivirals

Although DENV poses a significant health threat, there are currently no approved antiviral treatments for dengue infection. Nonetheless, researchers have investigated various strategies to develop antiviral agents targeting different aspects of the virus's lifecycle, including host attachment factors, viral proteins, and stages post-infection such as replication and maturation [37]. Additionally, several repurposed drugs with potential antiviral activity, including chloroquine, balapiravir, celgosivir, and lovastatin, have been evaluated in randomized blinded clinical trials. Despite these efforts, there is still no conclusive evidence demonstrating their effectiveness in preventing complications associated with dengue infection [7].

Dengue Vaccine

The production of vaccines has been an enormous challenge in dengue therapies owing to the problem of its four antigenically diverse serotypes, which might cause illness. The development of a DENV vaccine has been impeded by the complexity of the four serotypes (DENV-1–4) and the possible involvement of antibody-dependent enhancement in severe dengue. Currently, the only vaccine available is Dengavaxia (CYD-TDV), which has gotten clearance from both the FDA and the WHO. The vaccine is a recombinant live attenuated tetravalent immunization that was initially authorized by Sanofi Pasteur in 2015. Dengvaxia was cleared by the US FDA in 2019 for use in US territory [38]. Currently, it is registered in 20 countries. Currently conducting phase 3 investigations are two new live attenuated dengue vaccines, TV003 and TVOO5, produced by Takeda (Japan) and the National Institute of Allergy and Infectious Diseases, respectively. Tetravalent dengue (TDEN), dengue purified inactivated vaccine (DPIV), tetravalent DNA vaccine against dengue (TVDV), live attenuated vaccine (CYD-TDV), subunit vaccine (V180, cED III), inactivated vaccine (PIV), DNA vaccine (TVDV), and viral vector vaccines (CAdVax-Den) are among the additional vaccines that are reportedly undergoing trial and experimental phases [39].

Natural Medicine

Several plant-based compounds are currently employed in combating DENV infections owing to offer specific advantages over synthetic medications, such as being nontoxic, safer, and less damaging. The antiviral, larvicidal, and mosquito-repellent properties of natural medicines confer activity against viral mosquitoes.

Citrus limetta

It is a citrus fruit commonly known as "sweet lemon", belonging to the *Rutaceae* family. Its peels are a good source of nutrients like carbohydrates, protein, calcium, magnesium, glutamic acid, and aspartic acid [40]. The essential oils isolated from it exhibit mosquito-repellent properties while extracts from peels exert larvicidal activity against *A.aegypti* [41].

Carica papaya

It is a highly nutritious fruit belonging to the *Caricaceae* family. It contains constituents including papain and chymopapain, which possess antiviral, antifungal, and antibacterial properties. It also exhibits other beneficial properties such as antihypertensive, antifertility, hepatoprotective, anti-inflammatory, and anti-amoebic [42]. The extract obtained from its latex is responsible for larvicidal properties [43].

Kaempferia parviflora

It is an herbaceous plant, vernacularly known as black ginger, or krachai dum. It belongs to the family of *Zingiberaceae*. The active components have been shown to protect against various diseases such as inflammation, hypertension, neurological disease, and abdominal ailments. As per studies, it also exhibits larvicidal activities against mosquitoes [44].

Artemisia absinthium

It is a perennial shrubby plant, known by myriad names such as wormwood, absinthium, maderwood, bitterer beifuss, and wermkraut. It comes under the genus *Artemisia* and belongs to the *Asteraceae* family [45]. It possesses various properties like insecticidal, antifeedant, repellent, pupalicidal, and larvicidal. Therefore, it has been utilized to treat numerous diseases such as malaria, inflammation, allergy, hypertension, jaundice, and dengue [46].

Azadirachta indica

It is a medicinal plant commonly known as "neem", belonging to the *Meliaceae* family. It contains various chemical constituents including nimbin, nimbdin, gedunin, margolone, nimbolide, and azadirachtin. It is known for its various bioactive compounds, including flavonoids, catechins, gallic acid, saponins, and tannins. Numerous research works have confirmed that the plant demonstrates a variety of pharmacological qualities, such as anti-inflammatory, antioxidant, anti-cancer, and antidiabetic benefits [47]. The studies confirmed that neem oil exhibits, insect-repellent, larvicidal, and pupalicidal activity against *A.ageypti* [48].

WHO RECOMMENDATIONS

The WHO plays a pivotal role in regulating global efforts to combat dengue and mitigate its effects on public health. Effective control of the virus's transmission and prevention of its impact on areas affected necessitates teamwork and collaboration amongst many stakeholders. To combat dengue, WHO engages with a variety of organizations. Its initiatives cover a broad spectrum of actions, such as:

Vector Control

The World Health Organisation (WHO) supports Integrated Vector Management (IVM) as an avenue to curb the global epidemic of dengue fever. IVM implemented numerous attempts to reduce the spread of dengue such as insecticide spraying, reducing larval sources, and monitoring water storage practices.

Personal Safety Precautions

Personal protective measures aim to prevent mosquito bites and minimize exposure to disease-carrying vectors. A few typical personal safety precautions include utilizing insect repellents, donning protective clothing, using nets to repel insects, employing mosquito coils, and adding screens to doors and windows.

Eliminating Breeding Sites

Removing or emptying containers, tires, flower pots, and other objects that collect stagnant water can reduce mosquito breeding sites around homes and communities.

Seeking Medical Care

For prompt diagnosis and treatment, a person should seek medical attention if they have any signs of vector-borne disease, such as fever, recurrent vomiting, restlessness, joint pain, or muscle aches.

SURVEILLANCE AND MONITORING

To comply with epidemic trends throughout time and monitor dengue transmission, the WHO urges authorities to establish reliable monitoring platforms. The use of surveillance data aids in the identification of dengue outbreak areas of concern guides resource allocation and assesses the effectiveness of control measures [49].

CONCLUSION

This chapter provides a comprehensive overview of Dengue Virus (DENV), covering its structure, life cycle, diagnosis, and treatment. DENV, a member of the Flaviviridae family, consists of four serotypes and is transmitted primarily by Aedes mosquitoes. Understanding its structure and life cycle, including viral entry, replication, and release, is crucial for developing effective diagnostic and treatment strategies. Diagnosis often involves clinical evaluation, serological tests, and molecular techniques like PCR, enabling timely intervention. While supportive care remains the cornerstone of treatment for dengue fever, ongoing research into antiviral therapies and vaccine development offers hope for improved management and control of this significant global health threat.

REFERENCES

[1]   Malik S, Ahsan O, Mumtaz H, Tahir Khan M, Sah R, Waheed Y. Tracing down the Updates on Dengue Virus—Molecular Biology, Antivirals, and Vaccine Strategies. Vaccines (Basel) 2023; 11(8): 1328.
[http://dx.doi.org/10.3390/vaccines11081328] [PMID: 37631896]

[2]   Tuiskunen Bäck A, Lundkvist Å. Dengue viruses – an overview. Infect Ecol Epidemiol 2013; 3(1): 19839.
[http://dx.doi.org/10.3402/iee.v3i0.19839]

[3]   Vasilakis N, Cardosa J, Hanley KA, Holmes EC, Weaver SC. Fever from the forest: prospects for the continued emergence of sylvatic dengue virus and its impact on public health. Nat Rev Microbiol 2011; 9(7): 532-41.
[http://dx.doi.org/10.1038/nrmicro2595] [PMID: 21666708]

[4]   Monath TP. Dengue: the risk to developed and developing countries. Proc Natl Acad Sci USA 1994; 91(7): 2395-400.
[http://dx.doi.org/10.1073/pnas.91.7.2395] [PMID: 8146129]

[5]   Liu J, Tian X, Deng Y, *et al.* Risk factors associated with dengue virus infection in Guangdong Province: a community-based case-control study. Int J Environ Res Public Health 2019; 16(4): 617.
[http://dx.doi.org/10.3390/ijerph16040617] [PMID: 30791547]

[6]   Htun TP, Xiong Z, Pang J. Clinical signs and symptoms associated with WHO severe dengue classification: a systematic review and meta-analysis. Emerg Microbes Infect 2021; 10(1): 1116-28.
[http://dx.doi.org/10.1080/22221751.2021.1935327] [PMID: 34036893]

[7]   Wilder-Smith A, Ooi EE, Horstick O, Wills B. Dengue. Lancet 2019; 393(10169): 350-63.
[http://dx.doi.org/10.1016/S0140-6736(18)32560-1] [PMID: 30696575]

[8]   Available from: https://www.who.int/emergencies/disease-outbreak-news/item/2023-DON498

[9]   Available from: https://www.paho.org/en/topics/dengue

[10]   Available from: https://www.who.int/emergencies/disease-outbreak-news/item/2023-DON475

[11]   Available from: https://www.who.int/southeastasia/health-topics/dengue-and-severe-dengue

[12]   Shepard DS, Undurraga EA, Halasa YA. Economic and disease burden of dengue in Southeast Asia. PLoS Negl Trop Dis 2013; 7(2): e2055.
[http://dx.doi.org/10.1371/journal.pntd.0002055] [PMID: 23437406]

[13]   Available from: https://www.who.int/southeastasia/health-topics/dengue-and-severe-dengue

[14]   Nanaware N, Banerjee A, Mullick Bagchi S, Bagchi P, Mukherjee A. Dengue virus infection: a tale of viral exploitations and host responses. Viruses 2021; 13(10): 1967.
[http://dx.doi.org/10.3390/v13101967] [PMID: 34696397]

[15]   Chambers TJ, Monath TP. The flaviviruses: Detection, diagnosis and vaccine development. Elsevier 2003.

[16]   Diamond MS, Pierson TC. Molecular insight into dengue virus pathogenesis and its implications for disease control. Cell 2015; 162(3): 488-92.

[http://dx.doi.org/10.1016/j.cell.2015.07.005] [PMID: 26232221]

[17]   Xie X, Zou J, Puttikhunt C, Yuan Z, Shi PY. Two distinct sets of NS2A molecules are responsible for dengue virus RNA synthesis and virion assembly. J Virol 2015; 89(2): 1298-313.
[http://dx.doi.org/10.1128/JVI.02882-14] [PMID: 25392211]

[18]   Muñoz-Jordán JL, Laurent-Rolle M, Ashour J, *et al.* Inhibition of alpha/beta interferon signaling by the NS4B protein of flaviviruses. J Virol 2005; 79(13): 8004-13.
[http://dx.doi.org/10.1128/JVI.79.13.8004-8013.2005] [PMID: 15956546]

[19]   Roy SK, Bhattacharjee S. Dengue virus: epidemiology, biology, and disease aetiology. Can J Microbiol 2021; 67(10): 687-702.
[http://dx.doi.org/10.1139/cjm-2020-0572] [PMID: 34171205]

[20]   Zerfu B, Kassa T, Legesse M. Epidemiology, biology, pathogenesis, clinical manifestations, and diagnosis of dengue virus infection, and its trend in Ethiopia: a comprehensive literature review. Trop Med Health 2023; 51(1): 11.
[http://dx.doi.org/10.1186/s41182-023-00504-0] [PMID: 36829222]

[21]   Proutski V, Gould EA, Holmes EC. Secondary structure of the 3' untranslated region of flaviviruses: similarities and differences. Nucleic Acids Res 1997; 25(6): 1194-202.
[http://dx.doi.org/10.1093/nar/25.6.1194] [PMID: 9092629]

[22]   Polacek C, Friebe P, Harris E. Poly(A)-binding protein binds to the non-polyadenylated 3' untranslated region of dengue virus and modulates translation efficiency. J Gen Virol 2009; 90(3): 687-92.
[http://dx.doi.org/10.1099/vir.0.007021-0] [PMID: 19218215]

[23]   Cruz-Oliveira C, Freire JM, Conceição TM, Higa LM, Castanho MARB, Da Poian AT. Receptors and routes of dengue virus entry into the host cells. FEMS Microbiol Rev 2015; 39(2): 155-70.
[http://dx.doi.org/10.1093/femsre/fuu004] [PMID: 25725010]

[24]   Qi R, Zhang L, Chi C. Biological characteristics of dengue virus and potential targets for drug design. Acta Biochim Biophys Sin (Shanghai) 2008; 40(2): 91-101.
[http://dx.doi.org/10.1111/j.1745-7270.2008.00382.x] [PMID: 18235970]

[25]   Siqueira RC, Vitral NP, Campos WR, Oréfice F, de Moraes Figueiredo LT. Ocular manifestations in Dengue fever. Ocul Immunol Inflamm 2004; 12(4): 323-7.
[http://dx.doi.org/10.1080/092739490500345] [PMID: 15621872]

[26]   Raadsen M, Du Toit J, Langerak T, van Bussel B, van Gorp E, Goeijenbier M. Thrombocytopenia in virus infections. J Clin Med 2021; 10(4): 877.
[http://dx.doi.org/10.3390/jcm10040877] [PMID: 33672766]

[27]   Carod-Artal F. Neurological manifestations of dengue viral infection. Res Rep Trop Med 2014; 5: 95-104.
[http://dx.doi.org/10.2147/RRTM.S55372] [PMID: 32669894]

[28]   Sudulagunta SR, Sodalagunta MB, Sepehrar M, *et al.* Dengue shock syndrome. Oxf Med Case Rep 2016; 2016(11): omw074.
[http://dx.doi.org/10.1093/omcr/omw074] [PMID: 28031845]

[29]   Islam A, Cockcroft C, Elshazly S, *et al.* Coagulopathy of dengue and COVID-19: clinical considerations. Trop Med Infect Dis 2022; 7(9): 210.
[http://dx.doi.org/10.3390/tropicalmed7090210] [PMID: 36136621]

[30]   Shu PY, Chen LK, Chang SF, *et al.* Dengue virus serotyping based on envelope and membrane and nonstructural protein NS1 serotype-specific capture immunoglobulin M enzyme-linked immunosorbent assays. J Clin Microbiol 2004; 42(6): 2489-94.
[http://dx.doi.org/10.1128/JCM.42.6.2489-2494.2004] [PMID: 15184425]

[31]   Guzmán MG, Kourí G. Advances in dengue diagnosis. Clin Diagn Lab Immunol 1996; 3(6): 621-7.
[http://dx.doi.org/10.1128/cdli.3.6.621-627.1996] [PMID: 8914749]

[32] Jarman RG, Nisalak A, Anderson KB, *et al.* Factors influencing dengue virus isolation by C6/36 cell culture and mosquito inoculation of nested PCR-positive clinical samples. Am J Trop Med Hyg 2011; 84(2): 218-23.
[http://dx.doi.org/10.4269/ajtmh.2011.09-0798] [PMID: 21292887]

[33] Darwish NT, Alias YB, Khor SM. An introduction to dengue-disease diagnostics. Trends Analyt Chem 2015; 67: 45-55.
[http://dx.doi.org/10.1016/j.trac.2015.01.005]

[34] Yamada KI, Takasaki T, Nawa M, Kurane I. Virus isolation as one of the diagnostic methods for dengue virus infection. J Clin Virol 2002; 24(3): 203-9.
[http://dx.doi.org/10.1016/S1386-6532(01)00250-5] [PMID: 11856621]

[35] Muller DA, Depelsenaire ACI, Young PR. Clinical and laboratory diagnosis of dengue virus infection. J Infect Dis 2017; 215 (Suppl. 2): S89-95.
[http://dx.doi.org/10.1093/infdis/jiw649] [PMID: 28403441]

[36] Peeling RW, Artsob H, Pelegrino JL, *et al.* Evaluation of diagnostic tests: dengue. Nat Rev Microbiol 2010; 8(S12) (Suppl.): S30-7.
[http://dx.doi.org/10.1038/nrmicro2459] [PMID: 21548185]

[37] Lee MF, Wu YS, Poh CL. Molecular mechanisms of antiviral agents against dengue virus. Viruses 2023; 15(3): 705.
[http://dx.doi.org/10.3390/v15030705] [PMID: 36992414]

[38] Thomas SJ, Yoon IK. A review of Dengvaxia®: development to deployment. Hum Vaccin Immunother 2019; 15(10): 2295-314.
[http://dx.doi.org/10.1080/21645515.2019.1658503] [PMID: 31589551]

[39] Khan MB, Yang ZS, Lin CY, *et al.* Dengue overview: An updated systemic review. J Infect Public Health 2023; 16(10): 1625-42.
[http://dx.doi.org/10.1016/j.jiph.2023.08.001] [PMID: 37595484]

[40] Panwar D, Panesar PS, Chopra HK. Evaluation of nutritional profile, phytochemical potential, functional properties and anti-nutritional studies of *Citrus limetta* peels. J Food Sci Technol 2023; 60(8): 2160-70.
[http://dx.doi.org/10.1007/s13197-023-05743-x] [PMID: 37273556]

[41] Kumar S, Warikoo R, Mishra M, Seth A, Wahab N. Larvicidal efficacy of the citrus limetta peel extracts against indian strains of anopheles stephensi liston and aedes aegypti L. Parasitol Res 2012; 111(1): 173-8.
[http://dx.doi.org/10.1007/s00436-011-2814-5] [PMID: 22231268]

[42] Vij T, Prashar Y. A review on medicinal properties of Carica papaya Linn. Asian Pac J Trop Dis 2015; 5(1): 1-6.
[http://dx.doi.org/10.1016/S2222-1808(14)60617-4]

[43] Chandrasekaran R, Seetharaman P, Krishnan M, Gnanasekar S, Sivaperumal S. Carica papaya (Papaya) latex: a new paradigm to combat against dengue and filariasis vectors Aedes aegypti and Culex quinquefasciatus (Diptera: Culicidae). 3 Biotech. 2018; 8: 1-10.

[44] Panyakaew J, Sookkhee S, Rotarayanont S, Kittiwachana S, Wangkarn S, Mungkornasawakul P. Chemical variation and potential of Kaempferia oils as larvicide against Aedes aegypti. J Essent Oil-Bear Plants 2017; 20(4): 1044-56.
[http://dx.doi.org/10.1080/0972060X.2017.1377114]

[45] Szopa A, Pajor J, Klin P, *et al.* Artemisia absinthium L.—Importance in the history of medicine, the latest advances in phytochemistry and therapeutical, cosmetological and culinary uses. Plants 2020; 9(9): 1063.
[http://dx.doi.org/10.3390/plants9091063] [PMID: 32825178]

[46] Areshi S, Mashlawi AM, El-Shabasy A, Abdel Daim ZJ, Mohsen A, Salama SA. Larvicidal,

pupalicidal and adulticidal effects of *Artemisia absinthium* L. against dengue vector *Aedes aegypti* (Diptera: Culicidae) in Jazan region, K.S.A. Saudi J Biol Sci 2023; 30(12): 103853.
[http://dx.doi.org/10.1016/j.sjbs.2023.103853] [PMID: 38020224]

[47]   Islas JF, Acosta E, G-Buentello Z, *et al.* An overview of Neem (Azadirachta indica) and its potential impact on health. J Funct Foods 2020; 74: 104171.
[http://dx.doi.org/10.1016/j.jff.2020.104171]

[48]   Kaura T, Mewara A, Zaman K, *et al.* Utilizing larvicidal and pupicidal efficacy of *Eucalyptus* and neem oil against *Aedes* mosquito: An approach for mosquito control. Trop Parasitol 2019; 9(1): 12-7.
[PMID: 31161087]

[49]   Available from: https://www.who.int/emergencies/disease-outbreak-news/item/2023-DON498

CHAPTER 5

Zika Virus: Navigating the Public Health Landscape - Insights into Transmission, Symptoms, and Control Strategies

Tuhin James Paul[1], Ayushreeya Banga[1], Prabhjot Kaur[2], Rojin G. Raj[1], Gurmeet Singh[3] and Ashmeen Kaur[1,*]

[1] *Department of Pharmacy Practice, ISF College of Pharmacy, Moga, Punjab-142001, India*

[2] *Department of Food and Nutrition, Punjab Agricultural University, Ludhiana, Punjab-141004, India*

[3] *Department of Pharmaceutics, ISF College of Pharmacy, Moga, Punjab-142001, India*

Abstract: The Zika virus is characterized as an Arbovirus, more specifically as a member of the Flavivirus genus and the Flaviviridae family. Following its discovery in Africa in 1947, human cases of Zika virus infection remained few for more than five decades before spreading to the Americas and the Pacific. The structure of the Zika virus is common with Flavivirus but differs in the glycosylation site, the site is five amino acids larger and nearer to the immunodominant fusion which influences receptor interactions. The classification of Zika virus is based on genomic and phylogeny data, the most common Zika Virus strains are the ZIKV Asian strain and ZIKV Brazilian Strain. The main hosts for ZIKV are the non-human primates who undergo a sylvatic cycle with mosquito to spread the virus. Transmission can be zoonotic, sexual, arthropodal, and even maternofetal. Clinical features of the Zika virus include maculopapular rash/pruritis, conjunctivitis, fever, arthritis/myalgia, burning sensation in the extremities, retro-orbital pain, lymphadenopathy and rhinorrhea. By December 2021, there were recorded reports of Zika virus (ZIKV) transmission by mosquitoes in 89 countries and territories in five of the six WHO Regions, except the Eastern Mediterranean Region. There is a scarcity of accurate and up-to-date epidemiological data about the Zika virus. The annual incidence rate of the Zika virus (ZIKV) increased by an average of 72.85% every year between 2011 and 2015. From 20.25 per 100,000 in 2015 to 3.44 per 100,000 in 2019, there was a further drop. The bulk of ZIKV infections were detected in Latin America. While no definitive vaccines or drugs exist for Zika virus [ZIKV], promising candidates are undergoing clinical trials. Various antiviral strategies target viral and host proteins, while drug repurposing offers a faster, more cost-effective approach. WHO recommends viral control policies for the affected

* **Corresponding author Ashmeen Kaur:** Department of Pharmacy Practice, ISF College of Pharmacy, Moga, Punjab-142001, India; E-mail: ashmeenkaur100@gmail.com

regions. In this book chapter, one will learn about the characteristics, clinical features, epidemiology, prevention and guidelines on Zika Virus.

Keywords: Arbovirus, Arthropodal virus, Sylvatic cycle, Zoonotic transmission, Zika Virus [ZIKV].

INTRODUCTION

Aedes mosquitoes are vectors for the arbovirus, namely the ZIKV. This virus is an RNA virus, indicating that its genetic information is encoded on a solitary strand. It is classified under the Flavivirus genus and is a member of the Flaviviridae family. Mosquitoes may also transmit a variety of other flaviviruses, including dengue, Japanese encephalitis, West Nile, yellow fever, and Chikungunya, in addition to the Zika virus [2, 3]. It was discovered that a rhesus monkey discovered in 1947 in the African areas near Kampala, Uganda, was infected with the Zika virus. An arthropod that inflicts a bite on a vertebrate in order to transmit the virus is referred to as an arbovirus vector. There have been cases of nosocomial transmission *via* organ donation or bone marrow transfer, sexual transmission, and direct transmission from mother to child as nonvector arbovirus transmission mechanisms [4]. As of July 21, 2016, ZIKV infection was reported in sixty nations and territories. In 2018, India saw an outbreak of the Zika virus (ZIKV). ZIKV has been classified into two main lineages, African and Asian, based on their geographic origins according to phylogenetic study [2, 4, 5].

History and Discovery of Zika Virus

In 1947, a guard at the Uganda Virus Research Institute (previously known as the East African Virus Research Institute) spotted ill rhesus monkeys in the Zika jungle near Entebbe, Uganda. This was the first evidence of ZIKV. Later, Aedes africanus mosquitos in the same forest were proven to contain ZIKV, and testing on additional monkey species in the Zika forest confirmed that they were infected as well. There were no indicators of ZIKV infection discovered in serological studies of small animals observed in the Zika forest, including civets, giant pouched rats, squirrels, and tree rats. This study supports the hypothesis that primates, including humans and monkeys, are the principal vertebrate hosts of the virus. Six sentinel platforms with rhesus monkeys housed in cages were placed in Uganda's Zika Forest canopy in April 1947. On April 18, a rhesus monkey (number 766) held in a cage developed a temperature of 39.7°C. On the third day of the fever, the monkey's blood was collected, and the Swiss mice got it intraperitoneally, cerebrally, and subcutaneously, along with another rhesus monkey (no. 771). By day ten, every mouse that had been intracerebrally infected exhibited symptoms of disease, and their brains had been found to contain a filterable transmissible agent [6 - 8].

During the monitoring period, monkey number 766 only exhibited pyrexia; however, no additional abnormalities or increased body temperature were noticed in monkey number 771. Monkey No. 766 was infected with the ZIKV virus, or more particularly, the ZIKV 766 strain. During the convalescent phase, one month after the febrile episode and thirty-five days after inoculation, respectively, the serum from monkeys 766 and 771 neutralized this molecule. To isolate YFV, mosquitoes were caught in the Zika Forest in January 1948 [1]. Eighty-six Aedes africanus mosquitoes were collected after being spotted through the Seitz filter, and the mice were infected. One mouse died away on day six after immunization, while another felt unwell on day fourteen. The virus that was detected in Aedes africanus was identified as ZIKV [E/1 strain]. Rhesus monkey number 758 got a subcutaneous injection of the remainder of the Seitz filtrate. This monkey exhibited no indications of sickness [9 - 11]. However, two mice went away and one became unwell following an intracerebral injection of the monkey's blood; the sick monkey's serum included ZIKV [758 strain]. In response to the agent taken from its serum, rhesus monkey no. 758 developed neutralizing antibodies against the virus strains established from Ae. africanus (ZIKV E/1 strain) and rhesus monkey no. 766 (ZIKV 766 strain). The first human host of ZIKV, a 10-year-old Nigerian girl, was infected in 1954. Serum-neutralizing antibodies emerged in the two human ZIKV infections that survived, according to 1954 Nigerian research. In 1969, ZIKV was isolated from mosquitoes (Ae. aegypti) in Malaysia for the first time outside of Africa. Following that, in Indonesia's central Java area, the first human infections were detected in 1977 [6, 7, 12]. In 2007, there was an epidemic of the Zika virus on the isolated island of Yap in the western Pacific. Thirty-six years later, a big pandemic broke out in the South Pacific area of French Polynesia, with minor outbreaks emerging on other Pacific Islands. Most likely from the Pacific, the virus invaded Brazil between 2013 and 2015 and created a large outbreak that peaked in November 2015 before swiftly spreading throughout the Americas and Brazil, with some cases still circulating in the Pacific islands in 2016. The majority of Zika virus cases have been documented in Brazil's northeast and southeast. The Zika virus moved to North America in 2016 and was proven to be active in practically all Latin American and Caribbean nations as of January 2017. In November 2016, the Virus Research Diagnostic Laboratory in Ahmadabad, Gujarat, found the country's first Zika case. A few sporadic cases [in Gujarat and Tamil Nadu] and outbreaks of ZVD from the states of Rajasthan and Madhya Pradesh have occurred between 2017 and 2018. Real-time reverse transcriptase polymerase chain reaction (rRT-PCR) was utilized in October and November of 2021 in the Indian state of Uttar Pradesh to detect and validate over 100 Zika infections. There have been ZIKV virus outbreaks in two

Indian states: Madhya Pradesh (October–November 2018) and Rajasthan (September–October 2018). In the Madhya Pradesh and Rajasthan outbreaks of 2018, there were 159 and 127 ZIKV-positive cases, respectively [10, 13]. Table **1**, provides the chronology of the spread of Zika Virus among different countries mentioned in the table [6-14].

Table 1. Chronology of zika virus spread [14].

Year	Events	Area or Country	No. of Cases
2007	First large outbreak of ZIKV	Yap Island in the Federated States of Micronesia	49 confirmed and 7391 suspected cases
2013-2014	French Polynesia ZIKV outbreak, evidence of the Guillain–Barré syndrome; sexual transmission	French Polynesia, Easter Island, Cook Islands, New Caledonia	28 000–30 000 cases in French Polynesia; 1400 confirmed cases in New Caledonia
2015 -2016	ZIKV outbreak in the Americas	Brazil, Columbia, El Salvador, Mexico, Paraguay, Venezuela, Caribbean countries	440 000–1 300 000 estimated cases in Brazil; 51 473 suspected cases in Columbia
2016-2017	In 2016 ZIKV in continental USA. In 2017, First confirmed ZIKV outbreak in India	Florida and Texas. Confirm cases of zika virus report in Gujrat and Tamil Nadu.	4 cases in Florida. 3 cases Gujrat, 1 in Tamil Nadu.
2018	Biggest outbreak in India	Rajasthan, Madhya Pradesh	159 confirmed cases including 64 pregnant women in Rajasthan,130 cases in Madhya Pradesh

The urbanization of forest regions due to the expanding human population is the source of zoonotic infections like Zika virus. Furthermore, the ease and speed of mobility [roadways, trains, airplanes, and waterways] for both people and disease vectors adds to the speedy and broad spread of the sickness. A pair of ZIKV outbreaks in 2007 and 2013 opened a new chapter in the history of viral epidemiology. Numerous symptomatic patients and the fast spread of ZIKV across the Pacific Ocean islands to South America are features of these outbreaks.

Mosquitoes are the carriers of the ZIKV. Merely a tiny part of the several Aedes mosquito species—*Ae. aegypti, Ae. albopictus, Ae. hensilii, and Ae. polynesiensis*—from which ZIKV has been found has the capacity to function as efficient carriers of the virus.

Vectored by mosquitoes, ZIKV is an arthropod-borne virus, also known as an arbovirus. It is transmitted by two separate cycles: the sylvatic cycle, which includes humans and urban mosquitoes in cities transmitting ZIKV, and the urban cycle, which involves non-human primates and arboreal mosquitoes in forested regions spreading ZIKV. It is believed that two Aedes species mosquitoes—A. aegypti, which is distinguished by a bright lyre-shaped dorsal pattern with white bands on its legs, and *A. albopictus*, which is distinguished by a single longitudinal dorsal stripe with white bands on its legs—are the main carriers of ZIKV in an urban cycle. Between these two species, A. aegypti is the principal vector of the Zika virus epidemic. When non-human primates are missing, humans act as the major amplification hosts and transmission happens largely *via* urban and sylvan pathways [9, 15]. Because they are hematophagous arthropods, mosquitoes take up the virus *via* blood meals and continue to host it intact for the duration of their lives. During the succeeding blood meal, they transmit it to their target, the subsequent amplification host [4]. Fig. (**1**) provides a schematic flow of transmission for Zika Virus [4, 9-15].

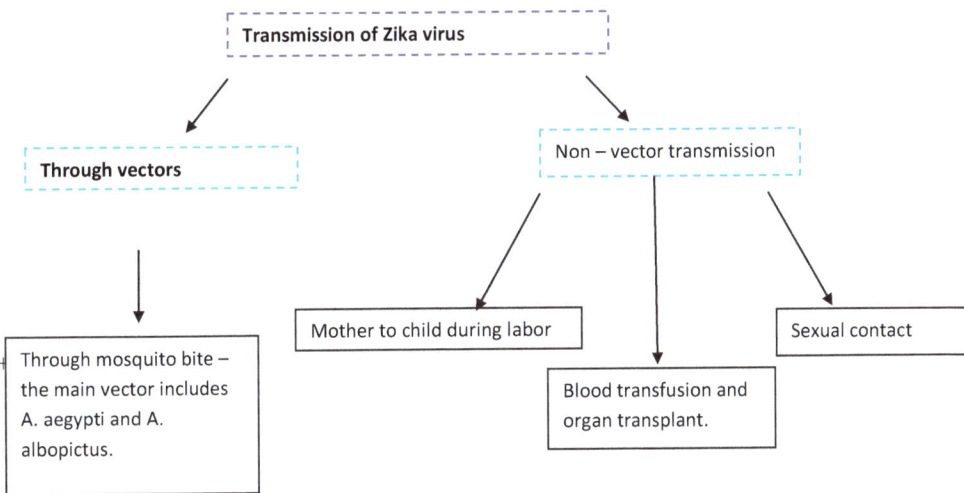

Fig. (1). Schematic Flow of Transmission [16].

A Zika virus infection may not display any symptoms at all, and its clinical signs and symptoms could range from mild to severe illness to sequelae. A maculopapular rash and/or conjunctivitis may occasionally accompany mild symptoms, which include pyrexia, asthenia, headaches, and myalgia along with a fairly modest infection. Congenital Zika syndrome is the term used to describe a range of congenital abnormalities that are suspected to be caused by the virus, such as microcephaly, Guillain-Barré syndrome (GBS), and neurological deficits. Zika is also suspected of causing miscarriages. Anorexia, vomiting, diarrhea, stomach aches, dizziness, leg discomfort, lymphadenopathy, and hypotension are some signs and symptoms [6, 17]. Fig. (**2**) describes the dynamics of Zika Virus transmission with two cycles (Sylvatic and Urban cycle) being shown by *A. aegypti* [18].

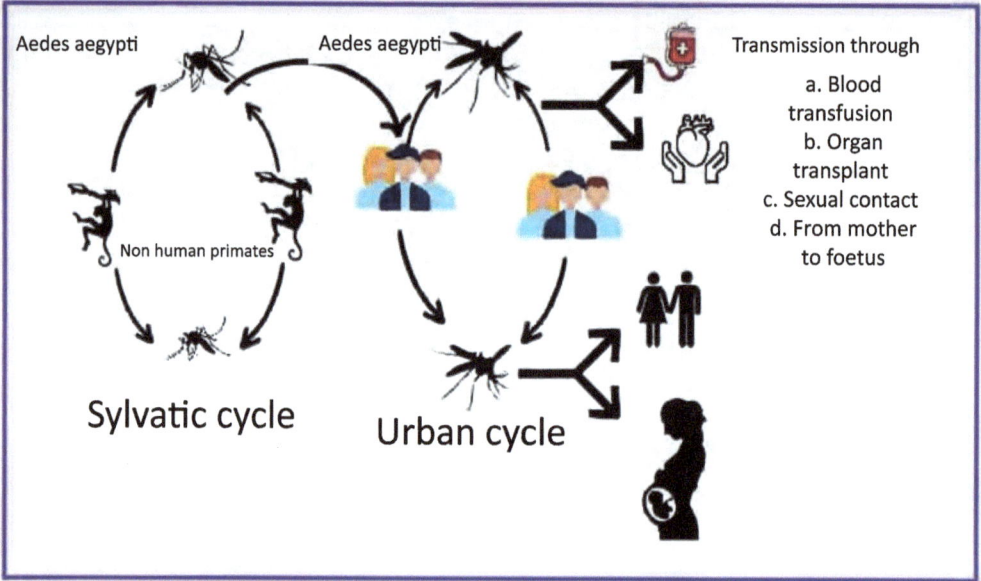

Fig. (2). Transmission Model [18].

Number of Cases of Zika Virus in Different Countries

An unexpected recurrence of Zika infections has been documented in over 84 countries globally. The sickness has raced across numerous continents, including Africa, South America, portions of Europe, Asia, and a Pacific Island. Brazil experienced recent outbreaks in 2015, and in 2016, the Americas witnessed outbreaks in 31 countries. EpiWATCH was designed by the Integrated Systems for Epidemic Response [ISER] at the NHMRC Centre for Research Excellence [22]. A "semi-automated epidemic observatory," EpiWATCH collects information on disease outbreaks and illnesses globally [7]. Table **2** describes the distribution of number of cases in countries such as the USA, Mexico, Thailand, *etc.* [4, 22]. Table **3** details the number of Zika Virus cases from 2016 to 2019 [4, 22]. Fig. (**3**) describes zika virus transmission cycles in urban areas [18].

Table 2. Distribution of number of cases in various countries [4].

Country	Number of Cases
United States	81115
Thailand	1044
Mexico	996
India	671

Table 3. Cases Reported from 2016-2019 [4].

-	2016	2017	2018	2019
Total no. of zika virus cases reported	81852	609	1800	15

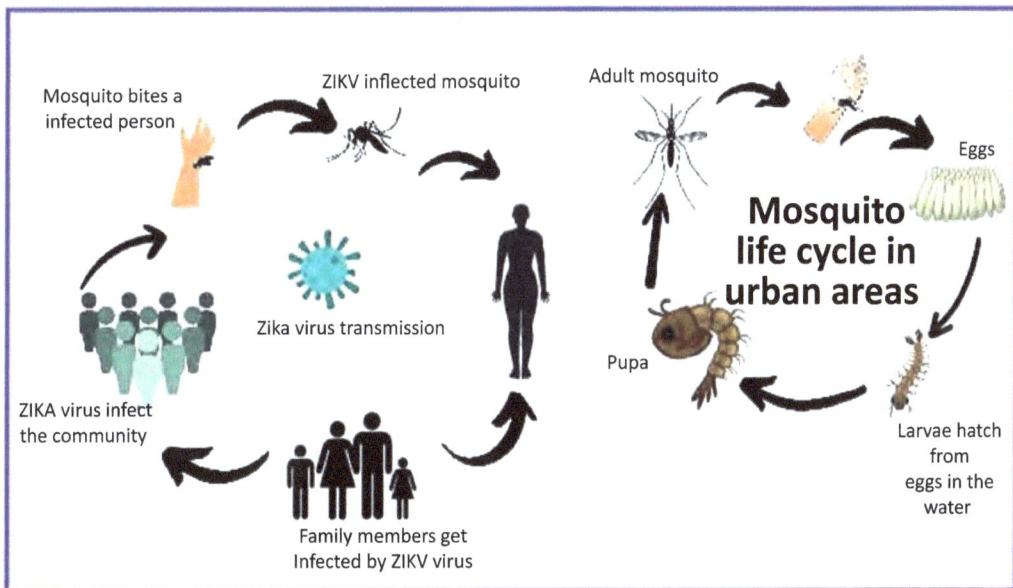

Fig. (3). Zika virus transmission cycle in urban areas [18].

Phylogeny of Zika Virus

Phylogenetic research of ZIKV has suggested the existence of two major viral lineages, African and Asian. ZIKV is a member of the Spondweni serocomplex. ZIKV and DENV are closely connected on the evolutionary tree, and they both cluster within the Spondweni group (Fig. **1**) [6, 18]. The Asian lineage, which includes strains found in Southeast Asia and the Pacific as well as current human ZIKV strains from the Americas, and the African lineage, which includes strains found in Central and Western Africa, are the two primary lineages of ZIKV strains. The polyprotein's 59 amino acids and 90% of its nucleotide sequence differ throughout the lineage [9].

Structure of Zika Virus

The virus ZIKV has an icosahedral structure and is spherical and encapsulated. The juvenile virus is more tightly spaced roughly 60 nm in diameter than the adult virus, which has a diameter of around 50 nm.

ZIKV is a member of the Flavivirus genus and a single-stranded positive-sense RNA virus with 11,000 nucleotides. ZIKV is a genome that is around 10.7 kb in length. It contains a single polyprotein and codes for roughly 10.2 kb. The seven non-structural proteins (Ns1 to Ns5), which are required for the virus's assembly and multiplication, and the three structural proteins (Capsid-C, Remembrance [membrane], Pram/M, and Envelope-E) make up the two major portions of the ZIKV genome. Encircling the ZIKV genome are the 5' and 3' untranslated regions [1]. Since it enhances viral admission into the host, glycoprotein E is a key target for antibodies. The stem-transmembrane domain pair and three extra-membrane domains known as ectodomains I, II, and III make up the four domains that make up the ZIKV E protein. The bigger E protein, which has a short extracellular domain, is situated atop the smaller M protein and makes up the bulk of the particle's surface [1, 19] stem-transmembrane domains and the region. A conserved region of the PrMprotein governs the maturation, egress, and secretion of viruses. It has been revealed that the capsid protein performs a vital role in viral assembly since it is the principal structural protein that interacts with the viral

DNA within the viral particle. For the virus to enter, translate, multiply, and become pathogenic, NS proteins are necessary. Their principal mode of action includes disrupting interferon [IFN], which assists the virus in avoiding the host's immune system I response [19, 20]. Because of its substantial function in immune evasion and replication, flavivirus NS1 is regarded as a pathogenicity factor and the most enigmatic protein. IFN I production is suppressed by ZIKV NS1 and NS4B, which initiates the autophagy pathway to remove NS2B and NS3 and end viral replication. It is known that by boosting Jak-1 degradation, NS2B3 [NS2B-NS3] inhibits the JAK-STAT pathway. The NS5 protein is the largest and most conserved of the flavivirus proteins, with roughly 900 amino acids. The NS5 protein comprises a methyltransferase for RNA capping and a polymerase for viral RNA synthesis NS2A is crucial for regulating virion morphogenesis and attracts viral RNA, the structural protein prM/E, and the viral NS2B/NS3 protease to the virion assembly site. Furthermore, it has been established that the flavivirus NS4A and NS4B proteins inhibit JAK/STAT [13, 19].

Immune Pathophysiology of ZIKA Virus

When a blood-feeding female injects the virus into a human's epidermis, arbovirus transmission occurs. Like other flaviviruses, ZIKV is spread *via* Aedes mosquito bites. Numerous cell types, including neurons, dendritic cells, and epidermal keratinocytes, have been confirmed to be targets of flaviviruses. ZIKV replication may be sustained in the human skin compartment. Infection led to time-dependent viral replication in fibroblasts, keratinocytes, and immature dendritic cells (iDCs) [14]. ZIKV initially interacts with cell receptors that are specific to distinct flaviviruses. ZIKV receptors include DC-SIGN [dendritic cell-specific intracellular adhesion molecule 3-grabbing nonintegrin] and the phosphatidylserine receptor proteins TYRO 3, AXL, TIM, and TAM. ZIKV may infiltrate fetal cells, monocytes, neural progenitor cells, NPCs, and macrophages owing to these receptors [21]. These receptors are critical for ZIKV infection in terms of adhesion, migration, replication, immune system evasion, cytokine production, and antigen signaling pathways. The fact that AXL improves human skin fibroblasts' sensitivity to ZIKV infection and replication implies that it is a crucial participant in the pathophysiology of viruses. AXL is overexpressed in glial cells and considerably expressed during neurogenesis in the developing human brain [14, 21]. Fig. (4) describes the structure of Zika Virus elucidating on its Proteinaceous nature [14, 21].

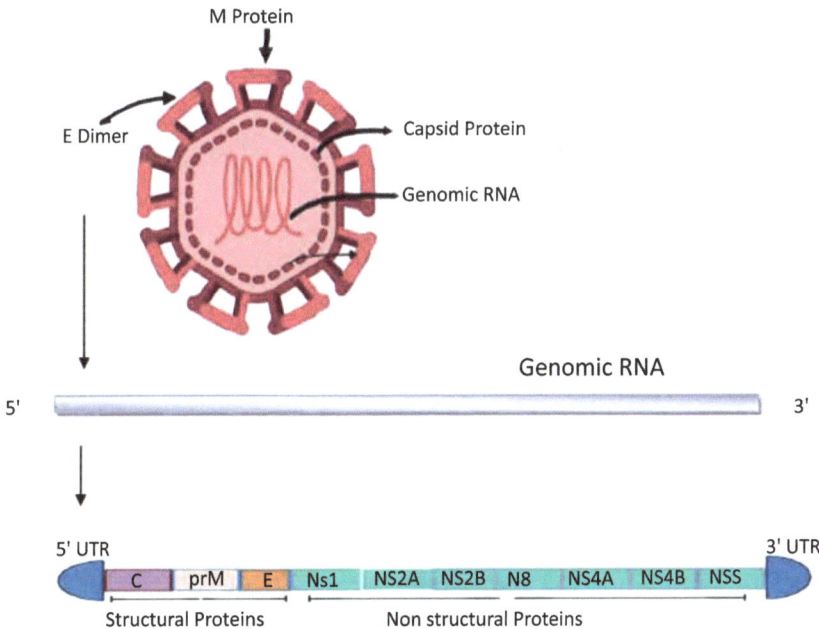

Fig. (4). Structure of Zika Virus [14].

The TIM family consists of three receptors: TIM-1, TIM-3, and TIM-4. Th2 cells and Th1 cells typically express TIM-3, whereas epithelial cells express TIM-1. Antigen-presenting cells are the only cells where TIM-4 is expressed. The PtdSer-dependent phagocytic clearance of apoptotic cells and the control of immunological responses are two of the multiple activities of TIM receptors. Members of the TAM receptor family, the protein tyrosine kinases referred to as TYRO3, AXL, and MER receptors, play a function in regulating immunological responses. TIM-1 and TIM-4 receptors appear to have a minimal role in ZIKV entrance into human skin cells; yet, investigations have revealed that both TIM and TAM family members collaborate in this process [14, 21, 22]. Fig. (**5**) describes the Immunopathophysiology of Zika Virus [14, 21]. Table **4** describes the protein present in a Zika Virus Structure.

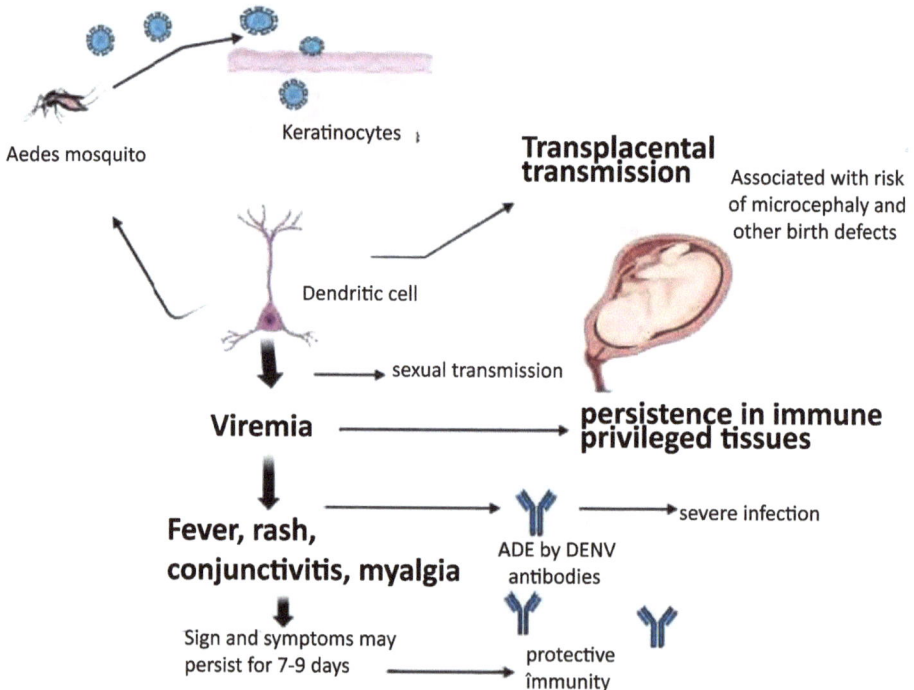

Fig. (5). Immunopathophysiology of Zika Virus [14, 21].

Table 4. Proteins In Zika Virus Structure [16].

C-Protein	Is Necessary for Viral Encapsulation
E-Protein	This Protein recognizes cellular receptors and entrance co-factors, and is the primary target for neutralizing anti-bodies.
NS1	NS 1 has a role in viral maturation, interaction with the prM and E proteins.

(Table 4) cont.....

NS2A	NS2A, a tiny hydrophobic protein found in the replication complex, has a function in influencing the host's anti-viral response.
NS2B	NS2B is a small transmembrane protein that functions as a chaperone for NS3, and its hydrophobic terminal domains attach the NS2B-NS3 Complex to the ER membrane.
NS3	Help in Viral replication

Clinical Features of Zika Virus

Zika virus infection typically causes a mild fever and flu-like symptoms for about a week. These include a low fever, a rash that starts on the face and spreads, red eyes without pus, muscle aches, joint pain in small joints, and headache. Some people may also have a cough, sore throat, vomiting, or nausea [16, 23]. Zika infection does not usually lead to severe illness or bleeding that requires hospitalization. The rash associated with Zika appears early in the illness, usually within the first week. It starts on the face and can spread to the rest of the body. Additionally, joint pain is a common symptom [16, 24]. Zika is a virus that may impact the nervous system; hence some individuals may have major neurological symptoms like facial paralysis, tingling or numbness, impaired hearing, inflammation of the brain and spinal cord, and weakness in the muscles [16, 25, 26]. Since the Zika virus has the ability to impact the nervous system, some patients may develop severe neurological symptoms including facial paralysis, tingling or numbness, hearing loss, inflammation of the brain and spinal cord, and muscle weakness. ZIKV does not cause major bleeding like dengue does, although it may create low blood platelets and blood in semen [27 - 29]. Despite being typically innocuous, ZIKV has killed individuals who already had health concerns and neonates who had microcephaly, a significant birth condition related with ZIKV infection in pregnant women. Guillain-Barré syndrome [GBS], an autoimmune nerve disorder that leads to weakness and paralysis, is another troubling outcome [29, 30]. Studies suggest a connection between ZIKV and GBS, with possible mechanisms involving immune reactions or changes in the virus itself. More research is needed to understand this link [29, 31]. The most concerning consequence is the surge in microcephaly cases in newborns exposed to ZIKV in the womb. These babies often have brain abnormalities and developmental delays. Even less severe infections might have long-term consequences [32]. Eye problems, for example, were observed in 30% of infants with suspected ZIKV infection. These findings underscore the necessity of more studies on the long-term repercussions of ZIKV infection, particularly for expecting women and their unborn children [33]. Understanding the full spectrum of complications is crucial for developing preventive measures and improving patient care. Table **5** given below provides an overview on the symptomology of Zika Virus across Age Groups and Pregnant woman [28, 31, 33].

Table 5. Zika Virus Symptomology across Age Groups and Pregnant Women [28, 31, 33].

Age Groups	Common Symptoms	Potential Complications
Paediatric	- Fever - Rash - Joint pain - red eyes [conjunctivitis] - Headache - Muscle aches - Vomiting and diarrhoea [less common]	-**Microcephaly:** smaller-than-expected head size in infants born to infected mothers, leading to developmental delays, vision and hearing problems, and seizures. - Other neurological problems
Geriatric	- Same general symptoms as adults [fever, rash, joint pain]	- Increased risk of **Guillain-Barré syndrome:** autoimmune disorder affecting nerves, causing muscle weakness and paralysis.
Pregnant Women	- Same general symptoms as non-pregnant adults [fever, rash, joint pain]	-**Transmission to fetus:** can cause birth defects like microcephaly and other neurological problems. - Even mild infection can have devastating consequences.

Co-Infections of Zika Virus

RT-qPCR is the main method used to detect coinfections, but these infections do not seem to cause different symptoms from single infections. In other words, people with coinfections experience the same signs and symptoms as those with only one infection [34]. Co-infections with Dengue [DENV], Chikungunya [CHIKV], and Zika [ZIKV] are becoming increasingly common, particularly in Southeast Asia and South America. Studies in India, Myanmar, Thailand, Ecuador, and the Colombian-Venezuelan border have all documented cases of co-infection with these mosquito-borne viruses. This is likely due to the shared vector [Aedes mosquitoes] and overlapping endemic areas. Even simultaneous co-infection by a single mosquito bite is possible. Understanding the clinical manifestations of these co-infections is crucial, as they can potentially impact disease severity and outcomes. To thoroughly comprehend the consequences of these co-infections on human health, additional investigation is necessary [35]. Zika, Dengue, and Chikungunya share overlapping symptoms, making diagnosis in endemic regions difficult. While all three can cause fever, rash, muscle aches, and joint pain, some differences exist. Dengue typically involves leukopenia and thrombocytopenia, while Chikungunya often presents with hepatomegaly and bleeding. Zika's most common symptoms are rash, joint pain, and fever. A study found only abdominal pain, leukopenia, and thrombocytopenia significantly differ between Zika and Dengue infections. Overall, accurate diagnosis relies on laboratory tests beyond just symptoms [36].

Complications of Zika Virus

While Zika virus often causes mild symptoms, it can lead to serious complications like Guillain-Barré syndrome and microcephaly in newborns exposed in the womb. This makes it crucial to avoid travel to Zika-endemic regions, especially when trying to conceive. Although most Zika infections show no symptoms, the potential for severe consequences underscores its dangers. Until treatments or a vaccine are developed, the best defence against Zika is preventing mosquito bites, particularly in endemic areas [37].

Animal and Human Models to Detect ZIKA Virus Epidemiology and Characteristics

Scientists lacked dependable animal models for Zika virus [ZIKV] infection prior to recent outbreaks. There were fears that because the main strain (MR766) was intended to grow in mouse brains, it wouldn't correctly mimic infections that occur normally. Recent efforts focused on new models using contemporary ZIKV strains. However, these models also showed limited disease signs in healthy mice. This resistance likely stems from ZIKV's ability to block the mouse immune response, something it can't do in humans. Despite challenges, some mouse models offer valuable insights. Studies with immune-compromised mice revealed eye disease and potential effects on the male reproductive tract. These models can help us understand specific aspects of ZIKV infection, even if they don't fully mimic human disease. The search for a perfect model continues, crucial for developing vaccines and treatments against this potentially dangerous virus [38]. Researchers are using non-human primates [NHPs] like macaques to understand how Zika virus [ZIKV] behaves and causes disease. Studies have infected pregnant and non-pregnant macaques with various ZIKV strains, observing symptoms, viral spread, and immune responses. Macaques typically experience mild symptoms like weight loss, rash, and elevated liver enzymes after infection. While symptoms may vary across studies, elevated liver enzymes seem consistent. Interestingly, ZIKV RNA was found in urine, saliva, and even the spinal cord, suggesting widespread dissemination. Tissue analysis revealed ZIKV presence in various organs, including the reproductive tract, intestines, and the brain, highlighting potential targets for the virus. Importantly, infected macaques also developed immune responses that could protect against future infections [39]. These findings solidify the use of macaques as valuable models for studying ZIKV infection and immunity. They give information on tissue tropism, long-term effects, and transmission of the virus, which opens the way to the construction of more effective vaccinations and medicines.

Current Treatment Strategies for Zika Virus

Despite the significant public health burden associated with Zika virus [ZIKV] infection, no specific antiviral agent has yet secured regulatory approval for this indication. Since acetaminophen and antihistamines increase the risk of hemorrhagic syndrome and Reye's syndrome, acetylsalicylic acid and nonsteroidal anti-inflammatory drugs (NSAIDs) cannot be used for symptomatic relief. Consequently, the development of effective and safe ZIKV antivirals remains a top research priority. Several promising avenues are currently being explored: 1) *De novo* drug discovery: This approach involves high-throughput screening of novel compound libraries to identify molecules that directly target and inhibit ZIKV replication. 2) Drug repurposing: Existing drugs with established safety profiles and efficacy against other pathogens are investigated for their potential to inhibit ZIKV replication. 3) Natural product exploration: The vast repository of bioactive compounds found in nature is being screened for potential antiviral activity against ZIKV [40]. 4) Antibody-based therapies: Efforts are underway to develop monoclonal antibodies or immune-based therapies specifically targeting ZIKV, aiming for viral neutralization and clearance [41]. These strategies have yielded a pipeline of promising antiviral candidates, some of which have progressed to early-stage clinical trials. However, further research and evaluation are necessary to identify potent, safe, and well-tolerated antivirals that can effectively combat ZIKV infection and its associated complications [9, 42].

Drug Repurposing in ZIKA Virus

Even if Zika virus [ZIKV] infection is typically asymptomatic, the devastating congenital brain abnormalities, neurological disorders, and infertility may underline the urgent need for effective prophylactic measures. Cao *et al.* emphasize the critical role of safe and well-tolerated drugs for prophylactic use, particularly among pregnant women [43]. Their proposed ideal candidate possesses specific characteristics ensuring fetal safety and efficacy: 1) Pregnancy Safety: Belonging to FDA pregnancy category A or B, minimizing potential risks to the developing foetus. 2) Oral Administration: Offering accessibility and convenience for widespread use. 3) Potent Antiviral Activity: Achieving sufficiently high blood concentrations to effectively combat ZIKV infection. 4) Limited Placental Transfer: For category B drugs, ensuring minimal passage to the fetus and prioritizing fetal well-being. Nitazoxanide emerges as a promising candidate due to its: 1) Oral Administration: Facilitating convenient and accessible delivery, 2) Pregnancy Category B: Possessing regulatory approval for use in adults and children over 1 year of age.,3) High Cmax: Reaching blood concentrations significantly exceeding the level required for complete viral clearance in *in-vitro* studies. While further research is necessary to fully evaluate the effectiveness and safety of Nitazoxanide in preventing ZIKV infection, particularly in pregnant women and their fetuses, its potential to meet these critical criteria warrants further investigation. If proven effective, Nitazoxanide could represent a valuable tool in safeguarding vulnerable populations from the devastating consequences of ZIKV infection [44, 45].

Researchers led by Barrows *et al.* [46] explored the potential of repurposing existing drugs to fight Zika virus [ZIKV] infection. They screened 774 FDA-approved medications, identifying 45 drugs that significantly inhibited ZIKV infection in human liver cells. Further evaluation narrowed this list to 24 promising candidates based on antiviral activity and clinical considerations [see Table **1** in the original text]. These drugs were then tested on various human cell types relevant to potential transmission routes and complications: **Cervical cells:** Representing the potential for sexual transmission prevention, drugs like mycophenolic acid and ivermectin completely blocked ZIKV infection at low concentrations. **Placental cells:** Simulating potential risks for pregnant women, several drugs, including mycophenolic acid, showed antiviral activity, with mycophenolic acid again being the most potent. **Neural cells:** Representing potential neurological complications, drugs like mycophenolic acid, ivermectin, and bortezomib exhibited antiviral effects, suggesting potential benefits for preventing or treating neurological damage. **Amniotic sac cells:** Representing potential risks to the developing foetus, mycophenolic acid, ivermectin, sertraline, and mefloquine showed strong antiviral activity, offering hope for protecting the foetus during pregnancy. These findings highlight the potential of repurposing existing drugs for ZIKV prevention and treatment, particularly considering the diverse range of affected cell types and the drugs' demonstrated effectiveness. Further research is needed to confirm safety and efficacy in humans, but this study offers a promising step forward in combating this potentially devastating virus [47].

Recombinant Reverse Technology Against ZIKA Infection

The advent of reverse genetic systems for the Zika virus [ZIKV] has offered scientists enormous tools to investigate the various subtleties of the virus's biology and pathogenesis in both *in vitro* and *in vivo* settings. Researchers have gotten a better grasp of the link between the virus and host and how it influences sickness symptoms by carefully manipulating the ZIKV genome to develop recombinant viruses with particular mutations. Furthermore, the discovery of innovative and more powerful strategies for halting and controlling ZIKV infections has been considerably facilitated by these reverse genetic approaches [48]. The value of these systems are considerably boosted by the generation of ZIKV replicons, or replicating-competent rZIKVs expressing reporter genes. This strong technology makes it simpler to discover antiviral medicines for ZIKV treatment [49]. This review meticulously analyses the three major strategies employed for generating rZIKVs: 1) **Infectious RNA transcripts:** This method entails the direct synthesis of infectious RNA transcripts from a full-length cDNA copy of the virus, 2) **Full-length infectious genomic cDNA clones:** This approach involves constructing an entire functional copy of the ZIKV's DNA in a laboratory setting. 3)**Infectious

Sub-genomic Amplicons [ISA]: This strategy utilizes smaller fragments of the ZIKV DNA to create replicating fragments. Similar to other flaviviruses, the presence of cryptic bacterial promoters within the viral genome has impeded efforts to maintain ZIKV cDNA sequences in bacterial hosts [50]. To overcome this instability, researchers have employed various strategies, including low-copy number plasmids, Bacterial Artificial Chromosomes [BACs], intron insertion, *in vitro* ligation of cDNA fragments, and *in vitro* assembly methods like Gibson assembly and CPEC [Competent Cell Electroporation of Plasmids]. While each approach offers unique advantages and disadvantages, a direct comparison to determine the optimal system for rZIKV generation and genetic stability remains elusive. Furthermore, the successful rescue of rZIKVs can be heavily influenced by biological factors, such as the chosen viral strain, and technical variables, like transfection methods. Finally, the generation of rZIKVs expressing reporter genes, combined with the development of ZIKV replicons, constitutes a vital toolkit for the identification of antiviral drugs against this significant human pathogen, readily adaptable to high-throughput screening settings. However, concerns regarding the stability of currently available reporter-expressing rZIKVs warrant further investigation and refinement. In conclusion, ZIKV reverse genetic systems have become cornerstones of virological research, empowering scientists to comprehend the virus, develop vaccines, and identify potential treatments. While certain challenges persist, these innovative techniques hold immense promise in the fight against this globally significant public health threat [51].

Surveillance System for Zika Virus

Zika virus disease [ZVD] surveillance primarily relies on healthcare providers reporting cases through a "notifiable disease" system. While seemingly straightforward, this passive approach presents significant challenges: Underestimation **of True Incidence:** A substantial number of ZVD cases remain undiagnosed or unreported, leading to an underestimation of the true burden of the disease. This "iceberg phenomenon" is evident in studies like Chevalier *et al.*'s, where blood donations revealed over 400,000 infections in Puerto Rico compared to 10,000 reported cases. **Data Integrity Concerns:** Incomplete reporting from private laboratories and lack of contextual patient information from public labs compromise data quality. **Variable Testing Practices:** Testing patterns are influenced by public awareness, healthcare access, and local transmission dynamics, introducing bias into surveillance data. **Circular Reporting:** Active surveillance triggered by reported cases can create a feedback loop, impacting data interpretation, **Misinterpretation Risk:** Subtle methodological nuances may be overlooked by policymakers and the public, leading to misinformed conclusions. Transitioning from passive to **population-based surveillance** offers a promising approach [52]. This involves testing representative samples, such as blood donors or prenatal care participants, regardless of individual healthcare decisions. Blind surveillance, where Zika status is unknown during testing, can further mitigate bias. Additionally, nationally representative surveys can provide valuable insights into the overall prevalence of the virus. Improved surveillance data accuracy will lead to More reliable trend analysis and comparisons: Enabling better understanding of ZVD transmission patterns and disparities across populations. Informed public health decisions: Facilitating optimal resource allocation and intervention strategies for effective disease control. While no solution is foolproof, transitioning from the current limitations to a more robust data-driven approach is crucial for effectively managing ZVD. By acknowledging the inherent challenges and embracing innovative solutions, we can gain a clearer picture of the disease and implement targeted measures to protect public health [53 - 56]. Table **6** gives a comparative analysis on Zika Virus Surveillance System [4, 26, 55].

Table 6. Zika Virus Surveillance system - A comparative analysis [4, 26, 55].

Country	Surveillance Systems	Key Features	Weakness
United States of America	- Passive and active surveillance - Mosquito trapping and testing - Case reporting from healthcare providers and public health labs - Laboratory testing of blood and other samples	- Robust system with multiple layers of data collection - Strong public health infrastructure - Emphasis on data quality and analysis	May miss mild or asymptomatic cases - Reliant on healthcare providers to report cases - Limited resources in some areas
Brazil	- Passive and active surveillance - Similar to US system, but with additional focus on vector surveillance - Community-based surveillance activities.	- Strong focus on early detection and outbreak response - Adaptable system to changing situations - large network of public health workers.	- Underreporting of cases due to limited healthcare access - Data quality issues in some areas - Challenges in rural and remote regions.
Uganda	-Primarily passive surveillance - Case reporting from healthcare facilities - Limited laboratory testing capacity	- Simple and low-cost system - Focus on early detection and containment - Strong community engagement	- High risk of underreporting - Limited data on asymptomatic cases - Difficulty in tracking transmission chains
India	-Evolving system, transitioning from passive to active surveillance - Case reporting from healthcare facilities and sentinel sites - Increased laboratory testing capacity	-Growing awareness and efforts to improve surveillance - Integration with existing disease surveillance systems - Focus on capacity building	- System is still under development - Limited data on geographic distribution and transmission patterns - Challenges in data collection and analysis.

WHO Recommendation

While Zika's sexual transmission is confirmed, its true impact on disease burden remains unclear. Nonetheless, prevention measures are crucial given ongoing circulation. Current guidelines by CDC and WHO recommend delaying pregnancy attempts after potential exposure: 6 months for men and 2 months for women [CDC] or 6 months for both [WHO]. However, this raises concerns for billions living in Zika-prone areas and frequent travellers. Considering the potential disruption to family planning and potential unintended consequences, are these recommendations optimal. Studies show varying Zika detection times in semen [up to 69 days] and vaginal fluids [up to 2 days], with documented sexual transmission up to 41 days. Recent research suggests infectivity in semen might be shorter than previously assumed, with only a small percentage containing live virus and shedding limited to 30 days. Given the declining virus circulation and limited evidence for extended semen infectivity, the authors propose revising current recommendations. They suggest a unified 2-month delay for both men and women after potential exposure, aligning with the observed infectivity window and potentially minimizing unnecessary disruption to family planning. This revised approach balances the need for caution with minimizing unnecessary restrictions, potentially benefiting individuals and public health efforts [57].

CONCLUSION

Zika virus has emerged as a serious global public health challenge over the past decade. Once considered a mild disease, the association of Zika infection with severe birth defects like microcephaly and neurological disorders changed our understanding of the virus's danger. This document provided a comprehensive overview of Zika virus, covering its discovery, structure, transmission, clinical manifestations, epidemiology, prevention and control strategies. Some key aspects summarized include the identification of Zika virus from sentinel monkeys in Uganda in 1947. Molecular studies showed it belongs to the Flavivirus genus and exists as African and Asian lineages. Zika is primarily transmitted by Aedes mosquitoes, predominantly A. aegypti, though emerging evidence suggests other modes like sexual and vertical transmission. While most infections are asymptomatic, common symptoms include fever, rash and joint pain. However, of grave concern are links to birth defects in infants born to infected mothers and neurological disorders like Guillain-Barré syndrome. The review outlined Zika's rapid global spread after initial outbreaks in the Pacific Islands and Americas. Over 84 countries have reported local transmission as of 2021. Surveillance data shows thousands of cases annually, predominantly in Latin America. However, underreporting is a challenge given many mild infections go unnoticed. Animal and human models discussed provided insights into Zika's propagation in the body and potential long-term effects requiring further study. No specific antiviral or vaccine currently exists for Zika. However, promising drug discovery approaches highlighted include repurposing existing medicines and natural compounds. Recombinant viral techniques and infection models are boosting research efforts. While symptomatic care remains the mainstay, preventive strategies focus on mosquito control and travel advisories. Robust population-based surveillance can better guide public health policies for this significant pathogen. In conclusion, ongoing multidisciplinary research holds the key to curbing Zika virus disease and its devastating consequences through the development of epidemiological insights, diagnostic tools, treatments and preventive measures.

REFERENCES

[1]   Shankar A, Patil AA, Skariyachan S. Recent perspectives on genome, transmission, clinical manifestation, diagnosis, therapeutic strategies, vaccine developments, and challenges of Zika virus research. Front Microbiol 2017; 8: 1761.
[http://dx.doi.org/10.3389/fmicb.2017.01761] [PMID: 28959246]

[2]   Rawal G, Yadav S, Kumar R. Zika virus: An overview. J Family Med Prim Care 2016; 5(3): 523-7.
[http://dx.doi.org/10.4103/2249-4863.197256] [PMID: 28217576]

[3]   Kamal R, Mukherjee D, Singh A. An outbreak of eye flu virus in india. Curr Drug Targets 2023; 24(17): 1293-7.
[http://dx.doi.org/10.2174/0113894501275247231129112022] [PMID: 38053356]

[4]   Pielnaa P, Al-Saadawe M, Saro A, et al. Zika virus-spread, epidemiology, genome, transmission cycle, clinical manifestation, associated challenges, vaccine and antiviral drug development. Virology 2020; 543: 34-42.
[http://dx.doi.org/10.1016/j.virol.2020.01.015] [PMID: 32056845]

[5]   Garg S, Garg G, Singh A. The resurgence of H3N2 in india: is it life-threatening? Curr Drug Targets 2023; 24(12): 931-3.
[http://dx.doi.org/10.2174/1389450124666230821092330] [PMID: 37605425]

[6]   Musso D, Gubler DJ. Zika Virus. Clin Microbiol Rev 2016; 29(3): 487-524.
[http://dx.doi.org/10.1128/CMR.00072-15] [PMID: 27029595]

[7]   Song BH, Yun SI, Woolley M, Lee YM. Zika virus: History, epidemiology, transmission, and clinical presentation. J Neuroimmunol 2017; 308: 50-64.
[http://dx.doi.org/10.1016/j.jneuroim.2017.03.001] [PMID: 28285789]

[8]   Sahoo S, Narang RK, Singh A. The marburg virus outbreak in west africa. Curr Drug Targets 2023; 24(5): 380-1.
[http://dx.doi.org/10.2174/1389450124666230213154319] [PMID: 36788691]

[9]   Baud D, Gubler DJ, Schaub B, Lanteri MC, Musso D. An update on Zika virus infection. Lancet 2017; 390(10107): 2099-109.
[http://dx.doi.org/10.1016/S0140-6736(17)31450-2] [PMID: 28647173]

[10] Yadav PD, Niyas VKM, Arjun R, et al. Detection of Zika virus disease in Thiruvananthapuram, Kerala, India 2021 during the second wave of COVID-19 pandemic. J Med Virol 2022; 94(6): 2346-9.
[http://dx.doi.org/10.1002/jmv.27638] [PMID: 35102566]

[11] Omosigho PO, John OO, Adigun OA, Hassan HK, Olabode ON, Micheal AS. The Re-emergence of Diphtheria Amidst Multiple Outbreaks in Nigeria. Infect Disord Drug Targets 2023.
[PMID: 38018182]

[12]   Kaur G, Singh A, Narang RK, Singh G. COVID-19 pandemic: age and temperature related effects. Coronaviruses 2021; 2(5): 11-9.
[http://dx.doi.org/10.2174/2666796701999200905095159]

[13]   Sapkal GN, Yadav PD, Vegad MM, Viswanathan R, Gupta N, Mourya DT. First laboratory confirmation on the existence of Zika virus disease in India. J Infect 2018; 76(3): 314-7.
[http://dx.doi.org/10.1016/j.jinf.2017.09.020] [PMID: 28988896]

[14]   Hamel R, Liégeois F, Wichit S, *et al.* Zika virus: epidemiology, clinical features and host-virus interactions. Microbes Infect 2016; 18(7-8): 441-9.
[http://dx.doi.org/10.1016/j.micinf.2016.03.009] [PMID: 27012221]

[15]   Kamal R, Mukherjee D, Khurana D, Singh A. Litchi: reason for the outbreak of acute encephalitis syndrome in bihar. Infect Disord Drug Targets 2024; 24(6): e170124225721.
[http://dx.doi.org/10.2174/0118715265276324231222113406] [PMID: 38243968]

[16]   Karkhah A, Nouri HR, Javanian M, *et al.* Zika virus: epidemiology, clinical aspects, diagnosis, and control of infection. Eur J Clin Microbiol Infect Dis 2018; 37(11): 2035-43.
[http://dx.doi.org/10.1007/s10096-018-3354-z] [PMID: 30167886]

[17]   Singh A, John OO, Bisola BB. Hand, Foot, and mouth disease outbreak what you need to know. infectious disorders-drug targets (formerly current drug targets-infectious disorders). 2023; 23(7): 77-81.

[18]   Vorou R. Zika virus, vectors, reservoirs, amplifying hosts, and their potential to spread worldwide: what we know and what we should investigate urgently. Int J Infect Dis 2016; 48: 85-90.
[http://dx.doi.org/10.1016/j.ijid.2016.05.014] [PMID: 27208633]

[19]   Mwaliko C, Nyaruaba R, Zhao L, *et al.* Zika virus pathogenesis and current therapeutic advances. Pathog Glob Health 2021; 115(1): 21-39.
[http://dx.doi.org/10.1080/20477724.2020.1845005] [PMID: 33191867]

[20]   Zanluca C, dos Santos CND. Zika virus – an overview. Microbes Infect 2016; 18(5): 295-301.
[http://dx.doi.org/10.1016/j.micinf.2016.03.003] [PMID: 26993028]

[21]   Barzon L, Trevisan M, Sinigaglia A, Lavezzo E, Palù G. Zika virus: from pathogenesis to disease control. FEMS Microbiol Lett 2016; 363(18): fnw202.
[http://dx.doi.org/10.1093/femsle/fnw202] [PMID: 27549304]

[22]   Sharma V, Sharma M, Dhull D, Sharma Y, Kaushik S, Kaushik S. Zika virus: an emerging challenge to public health worldwide. Can J Microbiol 2020; 66(2): 87-98.
[http://dx.doi.org/10.1139/cjm-2019-0331] [PMID: 31682478]

[23]   Nicastri E, Pisapia R, Corpolongo A, *et al.* Three cases of Zika virus imported in Italy: need for a clinical awareness and evidence-based knowledge. BMC Infect Dis 2016; 16(1): 669.
[http://dx.doi.org/10.1186/s12879-016-1973-5] [PMID: 27835966]

[24]   Salehuddin AR, Haslan H, Mamikutty N, *et al.* Zika virus infection and its emerging trends in Southeast Asia. Asian Pac J Trop Med 2017; 10(3): 211-9.
[http://dx.doi.org/10.1016/j.apjtm.2017.03.002] [PMID: 28442104]

[25]   Araujo AQC, Silva MTT, Araujo APQC. Zika virus-associated neurological disorders: a review. Brain 2016; 139(8): 2122-30.
[http://dx.doi.org/10.1093/brain/aww158] [PMID: 27357348]

[26]   Ozkurt Z, Cinar Tanriverdi E. Global alert: Zika virus-an emerging arbovirus. Eurasian J Med 2017; 49(2): 142-7.
[http://dx.doi.org/10.5152/eurasianjmed.2017.17147] [PMID: 28638259]

[27]   Foy BD, Kobylinski KC, Foy JLC, *et al.* Probable non-vector-borne transmission of Zika virus, Colorado, USA. Emerg Infect Dis 2011; 17(5): 880-2.
[http://dx.doi.org/10.3201/eid1705.101939] [PMID: 21529401]

[28] Musso D, Roche C, Robin E, Nhan T, Teissier A, Cao-Lormeau VM. Potential sexual transmission of Zika virus. Emerg Infect Dis 2015; 21(2): 359-61.
[http://dx.doi.org/10.3201/eid2102.141363] [PMID: 25625872]

[29] Lazear HM, Diamond MS. Zika virus: new clinical syndromes and its emergence in the western hemisphere. J Virol 2016; 90(10): 4864-75.
[http://dx.doi.org/10.1128/JVI.00252-16] [PMID: 26962217]

[30] Arzuza-Ortega L, Polo A, Pérez-Tatis G, *et al.* Fatal sickle cell disease and Zika virus infection in girl from Colombia. Emerg Infect Dis 2016; 22(5): 925-7.
[http://dx.doi.org/10.3201/eid2205.151934] [PMID: 27089120]

[31] Risk R. potential association with microcephaly and Guillain–Barré syndrome. update. 2016; 21: 5.

[32] Ventura CV, Maia M, Bravo-Filho V, Góis AL, Belfort R Jr. Zika virus in Brazil and macular atrophy in a child with microcephaly. Lancet 2016; 387(10015): 228.
[http://dx.doi.org/10.1016/S0140-6736(16)00006-4] [PMID: 26775125]

[33] De Paula Freitas B, de Oliveira Dias JR, Prazeres J, *et al.* Ocular findings in infants with microcephaly associated with presumed Zika virus congenital infection in Salvador, Brazil. JAMA Ophthalmol 2016; 134(5): 529-35.
[http://dx.doi.org/10.1001/jamaophthalmol.2016.0267] [PMID: 26865554]

[34] Carrillo-Hernández MY, Ruiz-Saenz J, Martínez-Gutiérrez M. Coinfection of zika with dengue and chikungunya virus zika virus biology, transmission, and pathology. Elsevier 2021; pp. 117-27.
[http://dx.doi.org/10.1016/B978-0-12-820268-5.00011-0]

[35] Suwanmanee S, Surasombatpattana P, Soonthornworasiri N, *et al.* Monitoring arbovirus in Thailand: Surveillance of dengue, chikungunya and zika virus, with a focus on coinfections. Acta Trop 2018; 188: 244-50.
[http://dx.doi.org/10.1016/j.actatropica.2018.09.012] [PMID: 30248317]

[36] Rothan HA, Bidokhti MRM, Byrareddy SN. Current concerns and perspectives on Zika virus co-infection with arboviruses and HIV. J Autoimmun 2018; 89: 11-20.
[http://dx.doi.org/10.1016/j.jaut.2018.01.002] [PMID: 29352633]

[37] Faluyi U, Obadare O, Sangem A, Onuegbu C, Medavarapu S. Complications associated with Zika Virus Infection: a systematic review study. Am Sci Res J Eng Technol Sci ASRJETS 2016; 24(1): 151-61.

[38] Morrison TE, Diamond MS. Animal models of Zika virus infection, pathogenesis, and immunity. J Virol 2017; 91(8): e00009-17.
[http://dx.doi.org/10.1128/JVI.00009-17] [PMID: 28148798]

[39] Dudley DM, Aliota MT, Mohr EL, *et al.* A rhesus macaque model of Asian-lineage Zika virus infection. Nat Commun 2016; 7(1): 12204.
[http://dx.doi.org/10.1038/ncomms12204] [PMID: 27352279]

[40] Haddad JG, Koishi AC, Gaudry A, *et al.* Doratoxylon apetalum, an indigenous medicinal plant from Mascarene Islands, is a potent inhibitor of Zika and dengue virus infection in human cells. Int J Mol Sci 2019; 20(10): 2382.
[http://dx.doi.org/10.3390/ijms20102382] [PMID: 31091703]

[41] Niu X, Zhao L, Qu L, *et al.* Convalescent patient-derived monoclonal antibodies targeting different epitopes of E protein confer protection against Zika virus in a neonatal mouse model. Emerg Microbes Infect 2019; 8(1): 749-59.
[http://dx.doi.org/10.1080/22221751.2019.1614885] [PMID: 31130109]

[42] Baz M, Boivin G. Antiviral agents in development for Zika virus infections. Pharmaceuticals (Basel) 2019; 12(3): 101.
[http://dx.doi.org/10.3390/ph12030101] [PMID: 31261947]

[43]   Narayanan R. Zika Virus Therapeutics: drug targets and repurposing medicine from the human genome. MOJ Proteomics & Bioinformatics 2016; 3(3): 00084.
        [http://dx.doi.org/10.15406/mojpb.2016.03.00084]

[44]   Devillers J. Repurposing drugs for use against Zika virus infection. SAR QSAR Environ Res 2018; 29(2): 103-15.
        [http://dx.doi.org/10.1080/1062936X.2017.1411642] [PMID: 29299939]

[45]   Zou J, Shi PY. Strategies for Zika drug discovery. Curr Opin Virol 2019; 35: 19-26.
        [http://dx.doi.org/10.1016/j.coviro.2019.01.005] [PMID: 30852345]

[46]   Barrows NJ, Campos RK, Powell ST, *et al.* A screen of FDA-approved drugs for inhibitors of Zika virus infection. Cell Host Microbe 2016; 20(2): 259-70.
        [http://dx.doi.org/10.1016/j.chom.2016.07.004] [PMID: 27476412]

[47]   Mottin M, Borba JVVB, Braga RC, *et al.* The A–Z of Zika drug discovery. Drug Discov Today 2018; 23(11): 1833-47.
        [http://dx.doi.org/10.1016/j.drudis.2018.06.014] [PMID: 29935345]

[48]   Atieh T, Baronti C, de Lamballerie X, Nougairède A. Simple reverse genetics systems for Asian and African Zika viruses. Sci Rep 2016; 6(1): 39384.
        [http://dx.doi.org/10.1038/srep39384] [PMID: 27991555]

[49]   Shan C, Xie X, Muruato AE, *et al.* An infectious cDNA clone of zika virus to study viral virulence, mosquito transmission, and antiviral inhibitors. Cell Host Microbe 2016; 19(6): 891-900.
        [http://dx.doi.org/10.1016/j.chom.2016.05.004] [PMID: 27198478]

[50]   Blaney J Jr, Hanson CT, Firestone CY, Hanley KA, Murphy BR, Whitehead SS. Genetically modified, live attenuated dengue virus type 3 vaccine candidates. Am J Trop Med Hyg 2004; 71(6): 811-21.
        [http://dx.doi.org/10.4269/ajtmh.2004.71.811] [PMID: 15642976]

[51]   Ávila-Pérez G, Nogales A, Martín V, Almazán F, Martínez-Sobrido L. Reverse genetic approaches for the generation of recombinant Zika virus. Viruses 2018; 10(11): 597.
        [http://dx.doi.org/10.3390/v10110597] [PMID: 30384426]

[52]   Hills SL, Fischer M, Petersen LR. Epidemiology of Zika virus infection. J Infect Dis 2017; 216 (Suppl. 10): S868-74.
        [http://dx.doi.org/10.1093/infdis/jix434] [PMID: 29267914]

[53]   Miller E, Hoschler K, Hardelid P, Stanford E, Andrews N, Zambon M. Incidence of 2009 pandemic influenza A H1N1 infection in England: a cross-sectional serological study. Lancet 2010; 375(9720): 1100-8.
        [http://dx.doi.org/10.1016/S0140-6736(09)62126-7] [PMID: 20096450]

[54]   Cowling BJ, Chan KH, Fang VJ, *et al.* Comparative epidemiology of pandemic and seasonal influenza A in households. N Engl J Med 2010; 362(23): 2175-84.
        [http://dx.doi.org/10.1056/NEJMoa0911530] [PMID: 20558368]

[55]   Piltch-Loeb R, Kraemer J, Lin KW, Stoto MA. Public health surveillance for Zika virus: data interpretation and report validity. Am J Public Health 2018; 108(10): 1358-62.
        [http://dx.doi.org/10.2105/AJPH.2018.304525] [PMID: 30138063]

[56]   Mercado-Reyes M, Acosta-Reyes J, Navarro-Lechuga E, *et al.* Dengue, chikungunya and zika virus coinfection: results of the national surveillance during the zika epidemic in Colombia. Epidemiol Infect 2019; 147: e77.
        [http://dx.doi.org/10.1017/S095026881800359X] [PMID: 30869010]

[57]   Vouga M, Musso D, Goorhuis A, Freedman DO, Baud D. Updated Zika virus recommendations are needed. Lancet 2018; 392(10150): 818-9.
        [http://dx.doi.org/10.1016/S0140-6736(18)31827-0] [PMID: 30146329]

CHAPTER 6

Understanding the H1N1 Pandemic: Characteristics, Global Impact, Treatment, and WHO Recommendations

Deepak Singh Bisht[1], Tuhin James Paul[2], Ayushreeya Banga[2], Amandeep Singh[3] and Pooja Chawla[4,*]

[1] *Department of Pharmaceutical Chemistry, ISF College of Pharmacy, Moga, Punjab-142001, India*

[2] *Department of Pharmacy Practice, ISF College of Pharmacy, Moga, Punjab-142001, India*

[3] *Department of Pharmaceutics, ISF College of Pharmacy, Moga, Punjab-142001, India*

[4] *University Institute of Pharmaceutical Sciences and Research, Baba Farid University of Health Sciences, Faridkot, Punjab-151203, India*

Abstract: Influenza viruses, especially the H1N1 type, can cause pandemics and seasonal flu epidemics, which makes them serious threats to public health. Global healthcare and financial systems are heavily burdened by these illnesses. Influenza viruses, especially those with swine origins, are highly adaptive and a constant threat, as demonstrated by historical outbreaks such as the Spanish flu of 1918 and the H1N1 swine flu pandemic of 2009. Comprehending the antigenic and genetic characteristics of H1N1 influenza is crucial for monitoring and formulating preventive measures, including immunization and antiviral drugs. To lessen the effects of influenza outbreaks, cooperation, vigilant worldwide surveillance, and preparedness for pandemics are crucial. In order to manage and stop the spread of H1N1, this abstract emphasizes the significance of continued study, teamwork, and preventive actions.

Keywords: Antigenic drift, Genetic reassortment, H1N1, Influenza, Pandemic, Swine flu.

INTRODUCTION

Influenza viruses are a major public health risk because they can cause pandemics as well as seasonal flu epidemics, which can happen at any time and especially during large crowds [1, 2]. These infections cause significant illness and death,

* **Corresponding author Pooja Chawla:** University Institute of Pharmaceutical Sciences and Research, Baba Farid University of Health Sciences, Faridkot, Punjab-151203, India; E-mail: pvchawla@gmail.com

putting a major strain on healthcare systems and economies worldwide [3, 4]. Annually, influenza viruses infect 20% to 30% of children and 5% to 10% of adults, according to the World Health Organisation (WHO), resulting in 3 to 5 million serious illnesses [5]. Seasonal influenza outbreaks cause more than 650,000 deaths worldwide each year [6, 7]. In the course of history, there have been numerous reports of influenza pandemics and epidemics of influenza. The most well-known of these is the Influenza A (H1N1) "Spanish flu" of 1918, which resulted in 500 million illnesses and 50-100 million deaths globally [8, 9]. H1N1 subtype viruses, most notably the H1N1 Swine flu, coexist with flu A (H3N2) viruses that first emerged during the 1968 epidemic [10]. Swine flu, a type of influenza A virus, infects the respiratory system causing fever, chills, and appetite loss, potentially reaching the lungs. This particular virus strain is commonly found in pigs worldwide, thus its common name, "swine flu." Humans, especially those living near pigs, are susceptible to contracting swine influenza viruses, which are usually zoonotic. However, unless there is a notable alteration in the antigenic properties of the virus through recombination, human-to-human transmission is typically ineffective [11]. 2009 saw the rapid global spread of a novel swine flu strain, H1N1, among humans, which prompted the World Health Organisation to proclaim a pandemic. Unlike typical swine flu, the 2009 H1N1 virus spread mainly between people through coughs, sneezes, or touching contaminated surfaces. The effective spread of the virus from human to human was made possible by a reassortment in the viral RNA structure. Maintaining alertness against these influenza pandemics is essential for preparing the world's health system. The dynamic nature and quick evolution of these viral illnesses exacerbate their worldwide impact, in addition to the ongoing threat of influenza pandemics. The 1918 influenza A (H1N1) "Spanish flu" and the 2009 H1N1 swine flu demonstrate how influenza viruses can genetically reassort and mutate to produce new strains that have the potential to spread to other areas and cause pandemics. The 2009 H1N1 virus rapidly spread over the globe, emphasizing the need for preparation and collaboration on a global scale in the fight against emerging infectious diseases. Outbreaks of influenza not only directly harm people's health but also place a significant burden on healthcare systems, lengthening hospital stays and consuming limited resources. Moreover, the economic impact of influenza-related illness and mortality on healthcare expenses and productivity is noteworthy. The fact that influenza has a dual cost on the health and financial systems highlights the urgent need for further study, monitoring, and the creation of potent vaccinations in order to lessen the disease's worldwide effects. The discovery of antiviral drugs, yearly immunisation campaigns, and public health awareness initiatives are all part of the complex efforts to prevent and control influenza. It is essential to continuously monitor influenza strains, especially those that have the potential to spread to humans, in order to detect infections early and take preventative action in a timely manner. The capacity of influenza viruses to adapt and spread effectively among humans presents an ongoing challenge, as evidenced by past pandemics, underscoring the significance of an active and cooperative worldwide strategy for pandemic preparedness [12, 13].

The Swine-Origin Antigenic and Genetic Properties

Influenza viruses that possess hemagglutinin (HA), which the human population is largely immune to, proliferate rapidly among individuals and can result in influenza pandemics. The genes responsible for attaching to and infecting cells (HA genes) in the most recent flu outbreaks of 1918 (H1N1), 1957 (H2N2), and 1968 (H3N2) can be traced back to bird flu viruses. All three viruses originated, either fully or partially, from nonhuman reservoirs. The first A(H11N1) influenza virus isolates from pigs were discovered in 1930 [14]. Significant antigenic similarity between the newly reconstructed human virus [15, 16] and the 1918 A(H1N1) virus points to a common ancestry [17]. For almost 70 years, between 1930 and the late 1990s, these traditional swine flu viruses spread only among pigs and did not change much in their structure (antigenically stable [18, 19]. A triple reassortant H3N2 (rH3N2) swine virus was circulating in swine populations across North America before or around 1998 [18, 19]. This virus arose from a mix of three influenza viruses: a classical swine flu virus, a modern human H3N2 flu virus, and an unknown subtype of bird flu from the American lineage. After the discovery of the rH3N2 virus, some scientists believe it mixed again with regular H1N1 swine flu, creating new versions of both H1N1 and H2N2 swine flu with a mix of genes from all three viruses [20, 21]. Human H1N1 flu strains gradually changed (drifted) away from the one that caused the devastating 1918 pandemic in the years leading up to the 1957 H2N2 outbreak [17, 22]. The A(H1N1) influenza strain that first infected humans reappeared in 1977 [23]. In light of the viruses included in the H1 component of the influenza virus vaccine, it was determined that eight updates were necessary between 1977 and 2009 [24]. The human H1N1 flu virus changed a lot over time, while the pig H1N1 flu virus stayed relatively the same. This big difference in how the viruses changed resulted in a major antigenic gap between human seasonal H1N1 and classical swine H1N1. Because of this, pigs are now a source of H1 viruses that could infect humans and cause a pandemic or serious respiratory outbreaks [25, 26]. Interestingly, Lys is present in all recognized human influenza viruses at site 627 in the PB2, which is a protein, but Glu^{627} is unique to influenza viruses that infect birds. All the 2009 A(H1N1) viruses studied so far have a building block called Glu at a specific location. The 1918 virus and the highly pathogenic H5N1 virus have both previously been connected to the PB1-F2 protein [27, 28]. The PB1-F2 protein, found in most influenza viruses, is cut short in all sequenced 2009

A(H1N1) viruses due to a stop signal at position 12 in its genetic code. The 2009 A(H1N1) virus also has a shorter NS1 protein due to a stop signal in its code. This missing piece called the PDZ ligand domain, is important for communication within cells and has been linked to the severity of some flu strains, like the 1918 H1N1 pandemic virus [29]. The research suggests the 2009 H1N1 virus might have unknown features that help it spread in humans. Existing flu vaccines target a protein on the virus's surface, but scientists are unsure how well these vaccines would work against this new strain. They studied the virus's antigenic properties and found it similar to other recent H1N1 strains that have occasionally jumped from pigs to humans in North America. Public health experts are concerned because this highly contagious virus has a unique genetic makeup and may not be well-controlled by current vaccines [30].

Etiology

The H1N1 swine flu virus is a tiny RNA virus with a genetic code around 13,500 units long. Despite its size, this code carries instructions for building 11 proteins, some crucial for infecting cells. Two key surface proteins, hemagglutinin (HA) and neuraminidase (NA), help the virus invade cells and spread. These proteins also help scientists distinguish between different flu strains, and the specific combination in H1N1 makes it unique. Changes in these surface proteins can allow the virus to infect people. The 2009 pandemic was caused by a special H1N1 strain with a unique genetic mix from four different flu sources: Eurasian swine flu, North American pig flu with bird genes, human flu with bird genes, and another North American swine flu. This genetic blend resulted in a highly contagious new virus [31 - 33].

Epidemiology

Swine flu has a long history, with the H1N1 strain being the dominant one for over 60 years after its discovery in pigs by American researchers in the 1930s. This flu not only affects pigs but can also jump between humans and pigs. Pork producers and veterinarians eventually recognized swine flu as a worldwide concern for pigs' health. The spread can be two-directional: pigs can catch flu strains from the people who care for them, and humans can become infected through close contact with pigs. In most cases, the virus had not spread beyond its initial location and had not caused outbreaks in new areas or infected people or pigs in other countries or continents. Regrettably, cross-species influenza virus transmission is always a possibility because of the swine flu virus's capacity for genetic diversity. Researchers came to the conclusion that the "2009 swine flu" strain, which started in Mexico, was referred to as the new H1N1 flu because it was mostly discovered to infect humans and displayed the surface antigens neuraminidase type 1 and hemagglutinin type 1. The 2009 H1N1 pandemic was caused by a unique flu virus with a mix of genes from human, bird, and swine flu strains. This new virus caused a global outbreak in 2009, with estimates of 43 to 89 million cases and 1799 deaths worldwide according to the CDC [34, 35]. Interestingly, the 2009 H1N1 virus was related to the devastating 1918 flu pandemic, which originated in pigs and jumped to humans. The 1918 flu strain still circulates in pigs, and occasional human infections from this lineage contribute to seasonal flu. While direct pig-to-human transmission is rare (only 12 cases reported in the US since 2005), pigs act as a reservoir for swine flu viruses, potentially reintroducing them to humans when our immunity weakens This is due to the potential retention of influenza virus strains in swine after these strains have disappeared in the human population [36, 37].

Pathophysiology

Swine flu, caused by the H1N1 virus, is a respiratory infection that primarily attacks the upper airways (like your nose and throat). In some cases, it can also spread to the lower airways (your windpipe and lungs). The recognized incubation period ranges from 1 to 4 days, with most individuals experiencing symptoms after an average of 2 days, though for some, it may extend to 7 days. Contagiousness in adults starts approximately one day before symptom onset, lasting for five to seven days. Swine flu can be contagious for longer in some people, especially children and those with weak immune systems. These folks might spread the virus for 10 to 14 days, compared to the usual 5-7 days in healthy adults. Typically, healthy individuals recover within three to seven days, but lingering symptoms such as coughing and malaise may persist for up to two weeks. Severe cases may necessitate hospitalization, potentially extending the infection period to nine or ten days. Swine flu symptoms like high fever, runny nose, and muscle aches are your body's way of fighting the virus. Serious side effects, including haemorrhagic bronchitis, viral pneumonia, or bacterial pneumonia, are more likely in pregnant individuals or those with heart or chronic lung disease. Complications may emerge 48 hours after initial symptoms. The virus replicates predominantly in the respiratory passages, peaking around 48 hours post-inoculation. Isolation of affected individuals for around five days is recommended [38]. H1N1 influenza, caused by the H1N1 influenza A virus, primarily spreads through respiratory droplets and can also be transmitted through contact with contaminated surfaces. The virus enters the respiratory tract, attaches to host cells, and undergoes replication, leading to an immune response and inflammation. Severe cases can result in pneumonia, acute respiratory distress syndrome (ARDS), and multi-organ failure. Risk factors include age, pregnancy, and underlying health conditions. The immune system produces specific antibodies, and recovery occurs once the infection is controlled. A comprehensive understanding of H1N1 pathophysiology is crucial for effective preventive measures, treatment, and public health interventions, encompassing vaccination, antiviral medications, hygiene practices, and social distancing [36].

Histopathology

Swine flu primarily affects the respiratory system, causing most of the symptoms to appear in the upper and lower respiratory tracts. While severe instances can clearly demonstrate pneumonia's pathologic changes, mild ones often only exhibit a few respiratory tract pathologic changes. Swine flu primarily attacks the cells lining your airways, both upper and lower. This damage can show up in a few ways: the cells themselves may detach and die, tissues under the lining can become red and swollen, and in rare cases, blood clots can form in smaller airways. In severe infections, the inflammation can become very serious, causing cells to shed in the smaller airways, bleeding in the airways, and even death of tissue in the walls of these smaller airways. In severe cases of swine flu pneumonia, the initial damage to airway cells can trigger an immune response, attracting white blood cells to the area. This damage to the lungs can then progress to widespread injury in the air sacs (alveoli), where oxygen exchange happens. Fluids, membranes, and even blood clots can form within these air sacs, further hindering oxygen intake. Additionally, tissue death and dead cells can accumulate, further compromising lung function. Long-term effects in some cases may include scarring, changes in cell types, and abnormal cell growth within the lungs. The diffuse alveolar damage and acute respiratory distress syndrome's fibroproliferative stage are characterized by these characteristics. Moreover, in several autopsy cases, bacterial coinfections were found. Staphylococcus aureus, methicillin-resistant Staphylococcus aureus obtained from the community, Haemophilus influenzae, Streptococcus pneumoniae, and Streptococcus pyogenes were the most extensively isolated bacteria.

Clinical Spectrum and Risk Factors Associated with H1N1 Swine Influenza

Swine flu (H1N1) symptoms can be all over the map. Some people get a mild flu, while others experience severe breathing problems or even death. This depends on a few things: your age, any other health problems you have, whether you've been vaccinated against the flu, and your body's natural defences against the virus The Centres for Disease Control and Prevention (CDC) reported that the 2009 H1N1 swine flu felt very similar to the seasonal flu for those infected. People with swine flu might experience a combination of symptoms including fever, chills, cough, sore throat, runny or stuffy nose, muscle aches, headache, dizziness, stomach pain, loss of appetite, and fatigue. This variability in symptoms makes diagnosis important, especially if you live in an area with a swine flu outbreak. While the

2009 H1N1 strain shared common flu symptoms, it also caused more vomiting and diarrhea than usual flu. Since these symptoms can occur with other illnesses, a detailed medical history is crucial, especially if you have been exposed to someone with confirmed swine flu or traveled to an outbreak area. In severe cases, the most common cause of death was respiratory failure. Other complications could include kidney failure, dehydration, severe low blood pressure (from vomiting and diarrhea), pneumonia leading to sepsis, high fever causing neurological problems, and electrolyte imbalances. Swine flu complications were more severe for certain groups. Young children under five and older adults over sixty-five were more likely to experience serious illness and even death. People with weakened immune systems due to medications, illnesses like cancer or autoimmune diseases, or even obesity were also at higher risk. Additionally, underlying health conditions like asthma, chronic lung disease, diabetes, or chronic heart problems increased the risk of severe complications. Pregnant women, particularly those in their third trimester, were also more susceptible to serious illness from swine flu.

Evaluation

Swine flu (H1N1) can mimic the flu or even cause pneumonia. If you have unexplained flu-like symptoms or pneumonia, especially in areas with swine flu outbreaks, doctors will consider it as a possibility. Regular checkups with blood tests and X-rays are helpful, but confirming swine flu requires a specific test. This usually involves a simple nose or throat swab. The rapid flu tests you might be familiar with won't always detect swine flu. Here's the key: if a test shows influenza A but not the markers for typical human flu, it suggests a new swine flu strain that might have jumped from animals (zoonotic). Antibody tests can sometimes confirm past zoonotic flu infections, but these can be unreliable due to similarities with human flu viruses. Public health labs are constantly vigilant, screening for new influenza viruses to prevent outbreaks.

Treatment/Management

Preventing swine flu is the first and best course of action in management, in particular, with the prevention of swine flu in pigs, the prevention of swine flu-to-human transmission, and the prevention of swine flu-to-human dissemination.

- Preventing Swine Flu in Pigs: The three main strategies for preventing swine flu in pigs are vaccination, herd management (not introducing influenza-carrying pigs into herds that have not yet been exposed to the virus), and facility management (using disinfectants and controlled temperature to suppress viruses in the environment). Strategies that exclusively focus on vaccination may not be sufficient since a major amount of the morbidity and death associated with swine flu is caused by secondary infection with other illnesses.

- Swine flu can jump from pigs to humans because pigs can catch flu viruses from both birds and people. This creates new flu strains. People who work closely with pigs, like farmers and vets, are most at risk of getting this swine flu directly. To protect themselves, they should wear face masks around pigs. The best way to prevent this spread in the first place is to vaccinate the pigs themselves. People who smoke or handle infected pigs without gloves or masks are more likely to catch swine flu because the virus can spread through hands touching contaminated surfaces and then the face.

- Swine flu spreads similarly to the seasonal flu. It can travel between people through contact with contaminated surfaces like hands, noses, and mouths, or by inhaling droplets from coughs and sneezes. While young children and the elderly may be contagious for a longer duration, most people spread the virus most easily within the first five days of feeling sick. To prevent the spread of swine flu, the Centers for Disease Control and Prevention (CDC) recommends frequent handwashing with soap and water or using alcohol-based sanitizers. Regularly disinfecting homes, hospitals, and public spaces with diluted bleach solutions can also help. If you live in an area with a swine flu outbreak and experience flu-like symptoms, it is important to avoid work and public transportation and get tested by a doctor as soon as possible to avoid further transmission.

- The H1N1 swine flu vaccine is the most well-known way to prevent swine flu. The FDA authorized the new swine flu vaccine in September 2009, and many studies done by the National Institutes of Health (NIH) showed that a single dosage produced enough antibodies to protect against the virus within 10 days. Those who have previously had a severe adverse reaction to an influenza vaccination should not take the vaccine. People who are moderately to critically unwell, particularly those with a fever, should be immunized once they have recovered or become asymptomatic.

The course of treatment for infected individuals is determined by the severity of their influenza symptoms. For mild to moderate cases, these can be managed at home with plenty of rest, fluids, and over-the-counter medications. This might include: Paracetamol, used for reducing fever, antipyretic for relieving nasal congestion and runny nose, pain relievers: NSAIDs or paracetamol for headaches and muscle aches. For severe cases, people with severe or worsening symptoms like trouble breathing, sepsis, or organ failure need immediate hospitalization, ideally in intensive care units (ICUs). Intravenous (IV) fluids are used to keep them hydrated, Electrolyte correction is done to restore imbalances in electrolytes; Antibiotics are used to fight any bacterial infections that may develop along with the flu. Mechanical ventilation: Machines are used to help people breathe if they have severe breathing problems (ARDS) due to the flu. This can be either noninvasive (through a mask) or invasive (through a tube placed in the windpipe), and ECMO (Extracorporeal membrane oxygenation): In most severe cases, especially with H1N1 ARDS, a special machine may be needed to oxygenate the blood outside the body. The antiviral medications zanamivir, oseltamivir, and peramivir, when provided within 48 hours of the beginning of symptoms, have been proven to help reduce or even prevent the effects of swine flu. Oseltamivir is known to cause skin issues, including sometimes severe skin conditions and occasionally brief neuropsychiatric episodes. Because of these potential side effects, oseltamivir is not recommended for use in the elderly or in persons who are more vulnerable to them. An egg allergy is the sole condition that precludes using zanamivir. The CDC began testing 1146 seasonal influenza A (H1N1) collected viruses on October 1, 2008, to determine their resistance to zanamivir and oseltamivir. Due to the body's hormonal, physiologic, and immune system alterations brought on by the H1N1 virus, pregnant women who get it are more likely to experience difficulties. For these reasons, the CDC advises vaccination against the swine flu virus for all expectant mothers. Neominidase inhibitors such as zanamivir and oseltamivir are antiviral drugs that can be used to treat swine influenza in pregnant women. It has been shown that taking these two medications within two days of falling ill maximizes their effectiveness [39 - 44].

Prevalence

The 2009 pandemic made the H1N1 virus, a subtype of influenza A virus, well-known. It causes seasonal flu outbreaks. The first cases of this unique strain were identified in the United States in April 2009, and it quickly spread over the world, infecting pigs, birds, and humans. The virus affected an estimated 284,400 individuals within its first year. Seasonal flu is now caused by a particular 2009 H1N1 virus strain. The A(H1N1) pandemic of 2009, which started in Mexico and spread to over 214 nations and territories, sickened previously healthy adults severely. Between 105,000 and 395,000 people are thought to have died. Even still, compared to some seasonal epidemics that can kill twice as many people, the pandemic turned out to be gentler. Following the 2009 pandemic, the World Health Organization (WHO) formed an international committee. They identified a major gap: the world wasn't ready for serious flu outbreaks or similar health emergencies. The committee called for several improvements: better overall health for people, stronger healthcare systems, economic development in poorer countries, building core public health capabilities, more research, and collaboration across different sectors.

CASES

2022-23

According to World Health Organisation, there was **10534** cases confirmed of Influenza A virus worldwide within 2022-23. There was a slight increase in cases of Influenza A virus.

2021-22

According to WHO estimates, there were only **8225** confirmed cases of influenza viruses globally in **2021-22**, with per month about 093 cases of influenza A (H1N1) . The cases slightly increase from the previous year.

2020-21

WHO data shows a big drop in confirmed influenza A (H1N1) per month cases between 2019-2020 (over 11,000) and 2020-2021 seasons (just 6,192).

2019-20

The World Health Organization (WHO) reported that during the 2019-2020 flu season, there were over 11,000 confirmed cases of influenza A (H1N1) per month and about 09 virus cases detected globally.

The above mentioned data from 2019-2023 is summarized in Fig. (**1**) [1].

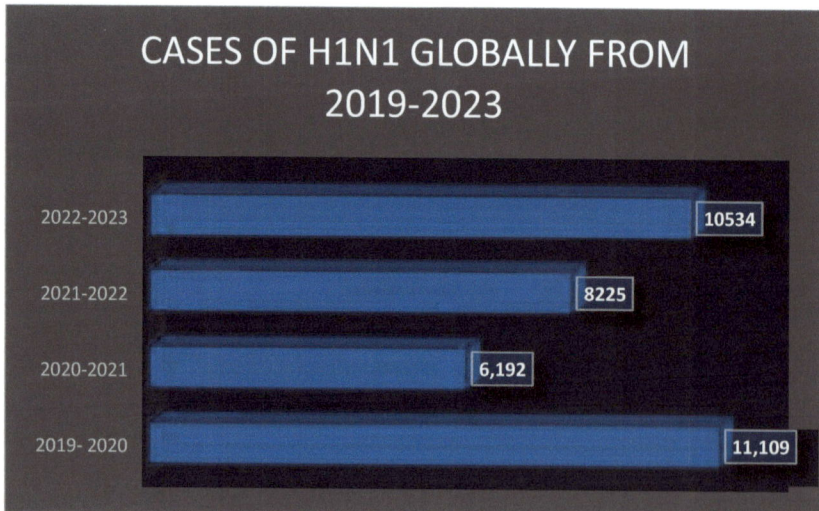

Fig. (1). Cases of H1N1 Globally From 2019-2023.

WHO Recommendation

The World Health Organization (WHO) maintains its current recommendations for public health measures and surveillance of seasonal influenza. This means there's no need for special screening of travelers entering neither countries, nor restrictions due to the ongoing interaction of influenza viruses between animals and humans. However, due to the constant evolution of influenza viruses, WHO stresses the importance of ongoing global surveillance. This vigilance helps to detect changes in the viruses circulating, whether related to their properties, how they spread, or how they affect human (and potentially animal) health. Timely sharing of virus samples is also emphasized to allow for proper risk assessment. The International Health Regulations (IHR) require notification for all human illnesses caused by a new influenza subtype. State Parties to the IHR (2005) shall immediately notify WHO of any laboratory-confirmed instance of recent human illness caused by influenza A virus with pandemic potential. Regardless of whether someone has symptoms, a complete epidemiological investigation is necessary if they test positive for, or are suspected of having, a novel influenza virus with pandemic potential, including variant strains. This examination should include a history of animal exposure, travel, and contact tracking, as well as the early detection of atypical respiratory episodes that may indicate person-to-person transmission. Clinical samples should be evaluated and sent to a WHO Collaboration Centre for further analysis. Based on existing knowledge, WHO does not propose any travel or trade restrictions for Germany. Travelers to countries with documented animal influenza epidemics should avoid farms, live markets, slaughterhouses, and surfaces polluted with animal faeces. Hand cleaning and adhering to appropriate food safety measures are recommended. The world has transitioned from phase 6 of influenza pandemic alert to the post-pandemic period. Views expressed by the Emergency Committee, convened by teleconference, highlight the global situation and reports from countries currently experiencing influenza. During the post-pandemic phase, the H1N1 virus is predicted to function similarly to seasonal influenza viruses, circulating for several years. Localized outbreaks of varying magnitudes may occur, as observed in New Zealand, necessitating vigilance, quick detection, treatment, and recommended vaccination. Globally, the levels and patterns of H1N1 transmission differ significantly from the pandemic, with out-of-season outbreaks no longer reported. Influenza outbreaks, including those caused by the H1N1 virus, now resemble the intensity typically seen during seasonal epidemics. The H1N1 virus no longer dominates, and a mix of influenza viruses is reported in many countries, akin to seasonal epidemics [45-47].

CONCLUSION

The complex nature of influenza, especially the H1N1 variant, calls for a worldwide coordinated approach to surveillance, prevention, and management. The 1918 Spanish flu and the 2009 H1N1 swine flu pandemic are two historical examples that highlight the influenza viruses' adaptability and highlight the continuous threat to public health. Given the potential for zoonotic transmission, the antigenic and genomic properties of influenza with swine origin highlight the need of tracking viral evolution. Vigilant surveillance is essential, particularly in populations where there is close contact with pigs. Understanding the genetic makeup and virulence aspects of H1N1 influenza can help develop tailored preventive strategies such as vaccination programmes and antiviral medications. Having a thorough understanding of the viral DNA enables proactive development of efficient defences. The epidemiology of H1N1, as shown by worldwide case counts, emphasises the necessity for ongoing surveillance by highlighting the fluctuating prevalence. The disease's pathophysiology, histology, and clinical spectrum provide insight into the variety of disease presentations that may occur. The elderly, young, and people with underlying medical issues are among the vulnerable populations. The changing environment necessitates continued study, global cooperation, and persistent pandemic readiness. The World Health Organisation emphasises global cooperation, quick reaction, and surveillance. Given the longevity of H1N1, we must maintain vigilant monitoring and take a proactive approach to controlling localised outbreaks.

REFERENCES

[1]   El-Kafrawy SA, Alsayed SM, Faizo AA, *et al.* Genetic diversity and molecular analysis of human influenza virus among pilgrims during Hajj. Heliyon 2024; 10(1): e23027.
[http://dx.doi.org/10.1016/j.heliyon.2023.e23027] [PMID: 38163192]

[2]   Available from: https://www.ncbi.nlm.nih.gov/books/NBK513241/

[3]   Garten RJ, Davis CT, Russell CA, *et al.,* Antigenic and genetic characteristics of swine-origin 2009 A (H1N1) influenza viruses circulating in humans. science. 2009; 325(5937): 197-201.

[4]   Lo CY, Tang YS, Shaw PC. Structure and function of influenza virus ribonucleoprotein. Subcell Biochem 2018; 88: 95-128.
[http://dx.doi.org/10.1007/978-981-10-8456-0_5] [PMID: 29900494]

[5]   Bailey ES, Choi JY, Fieldhouse JK, *et al.* The continual threat of influenza virus infections at the human–animal interface. Evol Med Public Health 2018; 2018(1): 192-8.
[http://dx.doi.org/10.1093/emph/eoy013] [PMID: 30210800]

[6]   Shi T, Arnott A, Semogas I, *et al.* the etiological role of common respiratory viruses in acute respiratory infections in older adults: a systematic review and meta-analysis. J Infect Dis 2020; 222 (Suppl. 7): S563-9.
[http://dx.doi.org/10.1093/infdis/jiy662] [PMID: 30849176]

[7]   Wen X, Huang Q, Tao H, *et al.* Clinical characteristics and viral etiologies of outpatients with acute respiratory infections in Huzhou of China: a retrospective study. BMC Infect Dis 2019; 19(1): 32.
[http://dx.doi.org/10.1186/s12879-018-3668-6] [PMID: 30621623]

[8]   Alfelali M, Khandaker G, Booy R, Rashid H. Mismatching between circulating strains and vaccine strains of influenza: Effect on Hajj pilgrims from both hemispheres. Hum Vaccin Immunother 2016; 12(3): 709-15.
[http://dx.doi.org/10.1080/21645515.2015.1085144] [PMID: 26317639]

[9]   Lamichhane PP, Samarasinghe AE. The role of innate leukocytes during influenza virus infection. J Immunol Res 2019; 2019: 1-17.
[http://dx.doi.org/10.1155/2019/8028725] [PMID: 31612153]

[10]   World health organization, Influenza (Seasonal), 2018. Available from: https://www.who.int/news-room/fact-sheets/detail/influenza-

[11]   Jilani TN, Jamil RT, Siddiqui AH. H1N1 influenza (swine flu). StatPearls. StatPearls Publishing 2019.

[12]   Rewar S, Mirdha D, Rewar P. Treatment and prevention of pandemic H1N1 influenza. Ann Glob Health 2016; 81(5): 645-53.
[http://dx.doi.org/10.1016/j.aogh.2015.08.014] [PMID: 27036721]

[13]   Xu X, Lindstrom SE, Shaw MW, *et al.* Reassortment and evolution of current human influenza A and B viruses. Virus Res 2004; 103(1-2): 55-60.
[http://dx.doi.org/10.1016/j.virusres.2004.02.013] [PMID: 15163489]

[14]   Khara NV, Kshatriya RM, Ganjiwale J, Lote SD, Patel SN, Paliwal RP. Lessons learnt from the Indian H1N1 (swine flu) epidemic: Predictors of outcome based on epidemiological and clinical profile. J Family Med Prim Care 2018; 7(6): 1506-9.
[http://dx.doi.org/10.4103/jfmpc.jfmpc_38_18] [PMID: 30613550]

[15]   Mukherjee R, Gunjan K, Himanshu K, Vidic J, Pandey RP, Chang CM. Advancing influenza prevention through a one health approach: A comprehensive analysis. Journal of Hazardous Materials Advances. 2024 May 1;14: 100419.

[16]   Keenliside J. Pandemic influenza A H1N1 in Swine and other animals. Curr Top Microbiol Immunol 2012; 370: 259-71.
[http://dx.doi.org/10.1007/82_2012_301] [PMID: 23254339]

[17]   Shope RE. Swine influenza. J Exp Med 1931; 54(3): 373-85.
[http://dx.doi.org/10.1084/jem.54.3.373] [PMID: 19869924]

[18]   Gorman OT, Bean WJ, Kawaoka Y, Donatelli I, Guo YJ, Webster RG. Evolution of influenza A virus nucleoprotein genes: implications for the origins of H1N1 human and classical swine viruses. J Virol 1991; 65(7): 3704-14.
[http://dx.doi.org/10.1128/jvi.65.7.3704-3714.1991] [PMID: 2041090]

[19]   Reid AH, Taubenberger JK. The origin of the 1918 pandemic influenza virus: a continuing enigma. J Gen Virol 2003; 84(9): 2285-92.
[http://dx.doi.org/10.1099/vir.0.19302-0] [PMID: 12917448]

[20]   Tumpey TM, García-Sastre A, Taubenberger JK, Palese P, Swayne DE, Basler CF. Pathogenicity and immunogenicity of influenza viruses with genes from the 1918 pandemic virus. Proc Natl Acad Sci USA 2004; 101(9): 3166-71.
[http://dx.doi.org/10.1073/pnas.0308391100] [PMID: 14963236]

[21]   Sheerar MG, Easterday BC, Hinshaw VS. Antigenic conservation of H1N1 swine influenza viruses. J Gen Virol 1989; 70(12): 3297-303.
[http://dx.doi.org/10.1099/0022-1317-70-12-3297] [PMID: 2558159]

[22]   Vincent AL, Lager KM, Ma W, *et al.* Evaluation of hemagglutinin subtype 1 swine influenza viruses from the United States. Vet Microbiol 2006; 118(3-4): 212-22.
[http://dx.doi.org/10.1016/j.vetmic.2006.07.017] [PMID: 16962262]

[23]   Karasin AI, Schutten MM, Cooper LA, *et al.* Genetic characterization of H3N2 influenza viruses isolated from pigs in North America, 1977–1999: evidence for wholly human and reassortant virus

genotypes. Virus Res 2000; 68(1): 71-85.
[http://dx.doi.org/10.1016/S0168-1702(00)00154-4] [PMID: 10930664]

[24]   Zhou NN, Senne DA, Landgraf JS, *et al.* Genetic reassortment of avian, swine, and human influenza A viruses in American pigs. J Virol 1999; 73(10): 8851-6.
[http://dx.doi.org/10.1128/JVI.73.10.8851-8856.1999] [PMID: 10482643]

[25]   Kilbourne ED, Smith C, Brett I, Pokorny BA, Johansson B, Cox N. The total influenza vaccine failure of 1947 revisited: Major intrasubtypic antigenic change can explain failure of vaccine in a post-World War II epidemic. Proc Natl Acad Sci USA 2002; 99(16): 10748-52.
[http://dx.doi.org/10.1073/pnas.162366899] [PMID: 12136133]

[26]   Webster RG, Bean WJ, Gorman OT, Chambers TM, Kawaoka Y. Evolution and ecology of influenza A viruses. Microbiol Rev 1992; 56(1): 152-79.
[http://dx.doi.org/10.1128/mr.56.1.152-179.1992] [PMID: 1579108]

[27]   Hay AJ, Gregory V, Douglas AR, Lin YP. The evolution of human influenza viruses. Philos Trans R Soc Lond B Biol Sci 2001; 356(1416): 1861-70.
[http://dx.doi.org/10.1098/rstb.2001.0999] [PMID: 11779385]

[28]   Bi Y, Yang J, Wang L, Ran L, Gao GF. Ecology and evolution of avian influenza viruses. Current Biology. 2024 Aug 5;34(15):R716-21.

[29]   Shinde V, Bridges CB, Uyeki TM, *et al.* Triple-reassortant swine influenza A (H1) in humans in the United States, 2005-2009. N Engl J Med 2009; 360(25): 2616-25.
[http://dx.doi.org/10.1056/NEJMoa0903812] [PMID: 19423871]

[30]   Conenello GM, Zamarin D, Perrone LA, Tumpey T, Palese P. A single mutation in the PB1-F2 of H5N1 (HK/97) and 1918 influenza A viruses contributes to increased virulence. PLoS Pathog 2007; 3(10): e141.
[http://dx.doi.org/10.1371/journal.ppat.0030141] [PMID: 17922571]

[31]   Zamarin D, Ortigoza MB, Palese P. Influenza A virus PB1-F2 protein contributes to viral pathogenesis in mice. J Virol 2006; 80(16): 7976-83.
[http://dx.doi.org/10.1128/JVI.00415-06] [PMID: 16873254]

[32]   Jackson D, Hossain MJ, Hickman D, Perez DR, Lamb RA. A new influenza virus virulence determinant: The NS1 protein four C-terminal residues modulate pathogenicity. Proc Natl Acad Sci USA 2008; 105(11): 4381-6.
[http://dx.doi.org/10.1073/pnas.0800482105] [PMID: 18334632]

[33]   He L, Zhang Y, Si K, Yu C, Shang K, Yu Z, Evidence of an emerging triple-reassortant H3N3 avian influenza virus in China. BMC genomics. 2024 Dec 26; 25: 1249.

[34]   Nogales A, Martinez-Sobrido L, Chiem K, Topham DJ, DeDiego ML. Functional evolution of the 2009 pandemic H1N1 influenza virus NS1 and PA in humans. J Virol 2018; 92(19): e01206-18.
[http://dx.doi.org/10.1128/JVI.01206-18] [PMID: 30021892]

[35]   Baudon E, Chu DKW, Tung DD, *et al.* Swine influenza viruses in Northern Vietnam in 2013–2014. Emerg Microbes Infect 2018; 7(1): 1-16.
[http://dx.doi.org/10.1038/s41426-018-0109-y] [PMID: 29967457]

[36]   Tapia R, García V, Mena J, Bucarey S, Medina RA, Neira V. Infection of novel reassortant H1N2 and H3N2 swine influenza A viruses in the guinea pig model. Vet Res 2018; 49(1): 73.
[http://dx.doi.org/10.1186/s13567-018-0572-4] [PMID: 30053826]

[37]   Hasan F, Khan MO, Ali M. Swine flu: knowledge, attitude, and practices survey of medical and dental students of karachi. Cureus 2018; 10(1): e2048.
[http://dx.doi.org/10.7759/cureus.2048] [PMID: 29541569]

[38]   Nelson MI, Souza CK, Trovão NS, *et al.* Human-origin influenza A(H3N2) reassortant viruses in swine, southeast mexico. Emerg Infect Dis 2019; 25(4): 691-700.
[http://dx.doi.org/10.3201/eid2504.180779] [PMID: 30730827]

[39]   Muthukutty P, MacDonald J, Yoo SY. Combating emerging respiratory viruses: lessons and future antiviral strategies. Vaccines. 2024 Oct 27;12(11):1220.

[40]   Nickol ME, Kindrachuk J. A year of terror and a century of reflection: perspectives on the great influenza pandemic of 1918-1919. BMC Infect Dis. 2019; 06; 19(1): 117.

[41]   Calore EE, Uip DE, Perez NM. Pathology of the swine-origin influenza A (H1N1) flu. Pathol Res Pract. 2011; 15; 207(2): 86-90.

[42]   Somerville LK, Basile K, Dwyer DE, Kok J. The impact of influenza virus infection in pregnancy. Future Microbiol 2018; 13(2): 263-74.
[http://dx.doi.org/10.2217/fmb-2017-0096] [PMID: 29320882]

[43]   Myers KP, Olsen CW, Gray GC. Cases of swine influenza in humans: a review of the literature. Clin Infect Dis. 2007; 15; 44(8): 1084-8.
[http://dx.doi.org/10.1086/512813]

[44]   Littauer EQ, Esser ES, Antao OQ, Vassilieva EV, Compans RW, Skountzou I. H1N1 influenza virus infection results in adverse pregnancy outcomes by disrupting tissue-specific hormonal regulation. PLoS Pathog 2017; 13(11): e1006757.
[http://dx.doi.org/10.1371/journal.ppat.1006757] [PMID: 29176767]

[45]   Available from: https://www.cdc.gov/h1n1flu/general_info.htm

[46]   Yang JR, Kuo CY, Yu IL, *et al.* Human infection with a reassortant swine-origin influenza A (H1N2) v virus in Taiwan, 2021. Virology Journal. 2022; 7; 19(1): 63.

[47]   Available from: https://www.who.int/emergencies/disease-outbreak-news/item/2023-DON486

Highly Pathogenic Avian Influenza A (H5N8) Virus: Structure, Case Studies and WHO Recommendation

Komal Mahajan[1], Diksha[2], Brajesh Kumar Panda[2], Prabhjot Kaur[3], Manish Kumar[1] and Amandeep Singh[1,*]

[1] *Department of Pharmaceutics, ISF College of Pharmacy, Moga, Punjab-142001, India*

[2] *Department of Quality Assurance, ISF College of Pharmacy, Moga, Punjab-142001, India*

[3] *Department of Food and Nutrition, Punjab Agricultural University, Ludhiana, Punjab-141004, India*

Abstract: The high transmissibility and pathogenicity of the H5N8 strain of the Avian Influenza virus pose serious threats to poultry populations worldwide. The introduction, traits, structure, history, features, prevalence, case studies, treatment, diagnosis, and WHO recommendations for H5N8 avian influenza are all covered in detail in this chapter. The virus mainly affects birds, resulting in severe symptoms like decreased egg production and respiratory discomfort. A multidisciplinary approach is required for diagnosis, which is essential for efficient management and surveillance. This approach includes clinical assessment, laboratory testing, and epidemiological investigation. Limited treatment options include antiviral drugs like zanamivir and oseltamivir, which are used off-label in birds. To track and contain zoonotic influenza outbreaks, the WHO recommends enhanced pandemic preparedness through risk assessment and intervention techniques, as well as international surveillance and cooperation.

Keywords: Avian influenza, Bird flu, Diagnosis, Epidemiology, H5N8, Poultry, Pathogenicity, Pandemic preparedness, Surveillance, Treatment, WHO recommendations, Zoonotic.

INTRODUCTION

Avian influenza is a highly transmissible illness that continues to spread throughout bird populations worldwide in poultry [1]. H5N8 is a very lethal strain of influenza A virus that is commonly referred to as bird flu in wild birds and

* Corresponding author Amandeep Singh: Department of Pharmaceutics, ISF College of Pharmacy, Moga, Punjab-142001, India; E-mail: ad4singh@gmail.com

Amandeep Singh (Ed.)

poultry [2]. Usually, H5N8 is not linked to humans. Viruses can jump to you in a few ways: by touching sick birds or their droppings, through contact with dirty surfaces, and even other methods. It is well known that H5N8 is very pathogenic in birds. Severe symptoms including respiratory discomfort, decreased egg production and elevated death rates can be experienced by infected chickens. Clinical symptoms in sick birds can include decreased egg production, and swollen eyes, neck, and head regions [3]. The influenza A virus, like its fellow A-type viruses, has a genetic instruction manual made up of eight pieces. This code tells the virus how to build at least 11 different tools it needs to function, including two important ones called hemagglutinin and neuraminidase. In avian species, HA and NA are categorized into 16 and 9 subtypes, respectively based on genetic variations. These two proteins play a crucial role in identifying different AIV serotypes. There are two main types of bird flu viruses: highly pathogenic (HPAIV) and low pathogenic (LPAIV). Scientists use a special test called the intravenous pathogenicity index (IVPI) to tell them apart. This test involves injecting the virus into chickens and observing how sick the birds get. By measuring the severity of the illness in chickens, the IVPI helps classify the virus as either highly pathogenic, causing severe disease and death, or low pathogenic, with milder effects or even no symptoms [4]. The H5N8 virus can manifest itself in a multitude of ways from asymptomatic and subclinical to highly lethal in some populations [5]. Numerous studies concerning wild birds are based on the discovery of dead animals. This virus is super deadly. It has a kill rate of at least 75%, which scientists can confirm through an IVPI test score of above 1.2.

Structure

The influenza A virus, including H5N8, possesses a complex structure comprising several key components:

Hemagglutinin (HA)

This protein is important for the virus to adhere to its target cells and effectively invade the host's body. In the case of this virus, the hemagglutinin subtype is represented as H5N8 and is contributed by the H5 type.

Neuraminidase (NA)

This enzyme assists in the ejection of the newly formed viral particles to the outer surface of the infected cells. With reference to H5N8, the neuraminidase subtype is N8.

Matrix Protein (M)

It is involved in the process of virus assembly and budding.

Nucleoprotein (NP)

Shelters the RNA virus genome and is required for replication and transcription.

Viral Polymerase Complex

This complex consists of PA, PB1, and PB2 which is required in the transcription process of the viral RNA genome.

Non-Structural Proteins (NS1 and NS2/NEP)

Such proteins assist in the control of viral reproduction rates and in the ability to avoid detection by the host's immune system.

The complete structure of H5N8 Virus is elucidated in Fig. (**1**) [1-5].

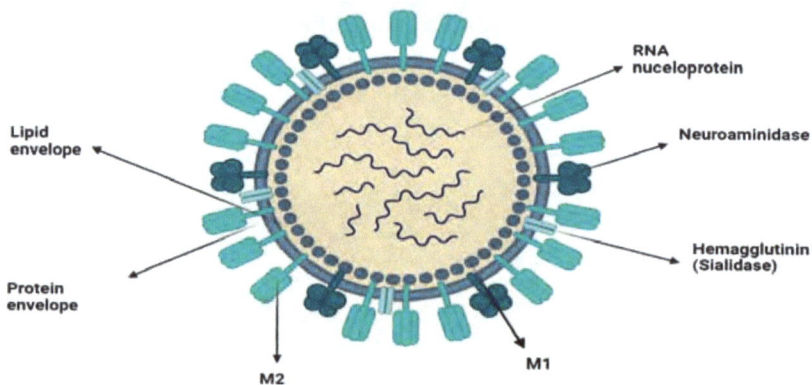

Fig. (1). Structure of H5N8 virus.

History

This new A (H5N8) strain was first reported in wild birds in Asia around 2010 and sub-sequentially emerged in domestic birds in China, South Korea, and Japan. It subsequently ventured into the European, Asian, and middle Eastern markets. Cross-migratory wild birds, which move from one continent to another such as in Egypt have also helped in the spread of the virus. H5N8 become notorious for its change and shifting that is sensitive to genetic reassortment which enhances its pathogenicity and its pattern of epidemic [6, 7].

Features

The H5N8 virus is characterized by its hemagglutinin subtype H5 and neuraminidase subtype N8. These proteins are essential for the virus's attachment to host cells and the release of new viral particles, respectively. Genetic analysis has identified H5N8 as a distinct subtype within the influenza A virus classification system [8, 9].

Prevalence

H5N8 avian influenza cases peaked in the US and Uganda in 2015, with high prevalence rates verified by RT-PCR and ELISA testing [10]. Birds that migrate such as Anas platyrhynchos and Anas Acuta, were important in spreading the infectious disease. The Three Egyptian isolates' genetic analyses identified a common ancestor of the highly virulent H5N8 avian influenza virus. A unique variation of the H5N8 virus spread through Europe in 2016, likely carried by migrating birds. This event highlighted the virus's ability to evolve and reassort, showcasing its potential for adaptation [11, 12]. 2014 saw the discovery of the Gs/GD H5N8 clade 2.3.4.4, which expanded throughout East Asia, Europe, and the western coast of North America. Concerns were expressed regarding the enhanced virulence of the H5N8 virus, particularly following fatal occurrences in birds such as Anser albifrons and sea eagles (Haliaeetus albicilla) [13]. In 2019, the infection also claimed a significant number of penguins lives. Epidemics arise as a result of interconnected global activity and the ability of infections to leap species [14]. Since the H5N8 virus first appeared in China in 2016 and 2018, there have been continuous global attempts to monitor and contain it [15]. H5N8 may be affected by the COVID-19 pandemic, and continued surveillance is essential to reducing its effects on the poultry sector in Europe, Central Asia the Middle East and Africa [16].

Case Studies

Between 1983 and 2023, numerous outbreaks of H5N8 avian influenza have been documented globally spanning countries such as Ireland, South Korea, Hungary, France, Nigeria, Uganda, Japan, Zimbabwe, South Africa, Saudi Arabia, India, Namibia, Iraq, China, Germany, Algeria, Afghanistan the United Kingdom, Japan, the United State and Argentina [16]. These outbreaks resulted in significant poultry culls and deaths with millions of birds affected. The measures including culling import bans and surveillance zones were implemented in various regions to control the spread of the virus. Additionally, the virus was found in both domestic and wild bird populations indicating its adaptability and widespread impact on avian species. The spread of H5N8 bird flu is raising new concerns about a wider outbreak. Scientists are now concerned that penguin populations in

Antarctica, far from the initial outbreaks, could also be affected. This highlights the virus's ability to travel long distances and the serious threat it poses globally [17].

From November 2020 to March 2021, Emi Yamaguchi and colleagues looked into H5N8 avian influenza outbreaks in 52 Japanese poultry farms. Larger flock sizes and closer proximity to water bodies increased infection risk in both layer and broiler farms, according to their simulation-based case-control study, which identified risk factors. Furthermore, the presence of waterfowl close to farms and the frequency of access by farm staff were linked to increased risk. These results highlight how crucial it is to put in place strong biosecurity protocols in chicken farms in order to stop the spread of extremely pathogenic avian influenza [18].

South Korea faced a harsh winter in 2020-2021 with outbreaks of a particularly severe type of bird flu (HPAI) – specifically different variations of the H5N8 strain. To track the spread and understand the virus better, a nationwide surveillance program was launched by scientists from the National Institute of Wildlife Disease Control and Prevention (NIWDC) under the leadership of Young Jae Si. This program involved collecting a massive number of samples (7,588) from various areas where wild birds live. 5.0% of the influenza A viruses that were isolated were HPAI H5N8 viruses which accounted for 38.5% of the isolates and were primarily detected in wild bird carcasses (97.3%). Novel HPAI genotypes resulting from genetic reassortment events were discovered through genetic analysis. Separate introductions of the G1 and G2 strains were made in Korea. While G2 emerged as the predominant strain that was consistently isolated, G1 viruses showed dynamic behaviour and produced a variety of sub-genotypes that were primarily isolated from clinical specimens [19].

In a study, three breeds of broiler chickens and ducks were used to examine the pathogenicity, immunogenicity, and potential for transmission of the H5N8 Highly Pathogenic Avian Influenza (HPAI) clade 2.3.4.4b virus by Nahed A. El-Shall and colleagues. Six log10 EID50 of HPAIV H5N8 were given directly to each group of ten chickens, Muscovy, Pekin, and Mallard ducks. On the day of infection, nine contact chickens were introduced to each group. Based on the mean death time (MDT) of 7.6 days, all of the infected chickens perished according to the results. With MDTs of 7 and 6 days, the mortality rates for Muscovy and Pekin ducks were 11.1% and 10%, respectively. Although they did not die, mallard ducks had a more severe clinical illness than Pekin ducks. Mallards displayed the most emotion [20]. A reassortant H5N8 avian influenza virus surfaced in Egypt towards the end of 2016. Researchers that studied the A/chicken/NZ/2022 strain genetically included Nahed Yehia. Using Madin-Darby canine kidney cells, they investigated its replication, pathogenicity, and viral load in comparison to earlier strains. The strain bore similarities to the 2.3.4.4b clade, which was identified in 2016 and demonstrated variation in H5N8 viruses in circulation. The cytopathic effect and high replication of A/chicken/Egypt/NZ/2022 suggested the possibility of field spread [21].

In France, 487 outbreaks of the highly pathogenic H5N8 avian influenza were reported during the winter of 2016–2017. A/decoy duck/France/161105a/2016 (H5N8), a particular strain was identified and examined using mule ducks. Three vaccines Vac1 derived from a different H5N8 strain, Vac2 containing a modified H5N1, and Vac3 containing a homologous H5 gene were tested to see if they could provide protection. The most effective treatment was Vac1 which eliminated shedding through the cloacal and oropharyngeal routes. Only cloacal shedding was eliminated by Vac3, whereas Vac2 only partially reduced it. These results shed light on the effectiveness of vaccinations in mule ducks, a crucial species in H5 HPAI outbreaks in France [22].

Concerning the dynamics of the Influenza A virus infection in ostriches, Celia Abolnik and colleagues studied this. One-week-old ostriches that were either infected with H7N1 LPAIV or belonging to clade 2. 3. 4. 4B H5N8 HPAIV were used and birds that were not challenged with any virus were grouped together. H5N8 HPAIV was pathogenic in exercising different levels of morbidity and mortality rates in contacts while H7N1 LPAIV did not cause severe pathogenicity in ostriches as evidenced by the mild symptoms. Tracheal shedding was the highest at 3-9 days post-inoculation in LPAIV and 8 days in HPAIV and surviving birds shed the virus beyond 14 days. Around and in feather pulp, the virus was found to be more and persisted up to 14 days local shedding correlated well with HPAIV. From day 7, the progression of a higher titer of antibodies provoked by HPAIV became evident. Altogether the susceptibility of the influenza A(H5N8) viruses isolated from Russia from 2014 to 2018 was tested by Svetlana V Svyatchenko and co-authors To eliminate non-specific inhibitors from H5N8-positive antisera, neuraminidase treatment was necessary. Resistance to adamantane was also observed with the M2-S31N strain only. In one strain, phenotypic analysis confirmed reduced oseltamivir inhibition. Clade 2. 3. 4. M2-S31N substitution was found to be commonly positioned in 4c viruses worldwide while 94% of clade 2. 3. 4. 4b virus was S31 M2 genotype positive. No or minimal resistance to neuraminidase inhibitors or amino-acid positions related to baloxavir was identified in most of the viruses. However, the analysed viruses did not possess the NA-N293/294S substitution, so it is important to remark. In epidemiological surveillance, this work highlights that influenza A(H5N8) viruses are not frequently reported to have decreased oseltamivir inhibition due to NA-N293/294S substitution [23, 24].

Mahmoud Ibrahim and associates sampled HPAI H5N8 viruses from chickens and geese between 2018 and 2019 in relation to clade-2. 3. 4. 4b. Umbach and the team produced a reassortant virus-containing monovalent and bivalent vaccines. In respective SPF chickens, the efficacy and safety profiles were evaluated. Full clinical protection against HPAI H5N8 and H5N1 was achieved with both vaccinations within two weeks with protective antibody titters. By day three post-infection, the bivalent vaccine divested HPAI H5N8 shedding completely while the shedding of HPAI H5N1 was substantially reduced by the bivalent vaccine. These results justify the use of a bivalent vaccine in the vaccination programs in endemic countries in order to show that it is effective in the protection of the chickens and the reduction of virus shedding. In Egypt, highly pathogenic H5N1 (clade 2. 2. 1) and low pathogenic H9N2 (G1-B lineage) avian influenza viruses were found to be common by Ahmad *et al.* Nonetheless, HP H5N2 reassortants with H9N2 viruses came out for the first time in 2016 due to the incursion of HPAIV H5N8 (Clade 2. 3. 4. 4b). This was done through tests conducted on 37 flocks, which indicated that 21 of them had HP H5N8 while 2 flocks also tested positive for H9N2. HA proteins of new Egyptian sequences had fewer mutations than the prior sequences seen in HA; nevertheless, M2 and NA proteins reflected some substitutions associated with resistance to amantadine and oseltamivir. At least seven HPAI H5Nx genotypes have been identified since 2016 due to the reassortment analysis of the Egyptian whole genome sequences wild bird origin has been suggested for internal gene segments. The mechanistic details remained uncertain because only a few partial genomes suggested annual replacement patterns of HP H5Nx genotypes while some genotypes seemed to convey selective benefits [25, 26].

Between January 2016 and December 2017, Awad Shehata A examined respiratory disorders and death rates in 50 poultry farms including 11 commercial layer poultry farms and 39 broiler poultry farms. Others that received attention include Greenfinch, Bluebird, and Quail samples. 64. 1% of broiler farms were tested through PCR screening for single virus infections; the most circulating viruses detected were New Castle disease (ND) at 33. 3% and H9N2 at 20. 5%, H5N1 at 7. 7% and H5N8 at 2. 7%. Also highlighted was co-infection with more than one virus and the most common virus combination was H9N2/ND (7. 7%). The only single infections were H5N1 and ILT with a prevalence rate of 18. 1% each, while H9N2/ND was the most prevalent at 27. 3%. Two samples of wild birds and one quail farm were both positive for H5N8. As expected, H5N8 and H5N1 sequences were identified to be grouped within the 2. 3. 4. 4 and 2. 2. 1. According to molecular data, they were divided into 2 clades, respectively. Surprisingly, chicken H5N8 was less antigenically related to AI H5N1 clades and this is manifested by the amino acid changes observed in the chicken H5N8 as compared to wild birds. The study calls for a shift of vaccination in Egypt and the incorporation of strict bio-security measures as it ascribes the formation of the possible AI epidemic strains due to a triple combination of H5N1, H9N2, and H5N8 [27].

Treatment

The approach to treating H5N8 infection in humans aligns with that of other influenza subtypes. Administering antiviral medications like zanamivir (Relenza) or oseltamivir (Tamiflu) within 48 hours of symptom onset can effectively reduce the severity and duration of the illness [28]. Table **1** provides an overview of the treatment of H5N8 avian influenza virus [29-34].

Table 1. Treatment of H5N8 avian influenza, along with their respective categories [29 - 34].

Drug	Category of the Drug	Use	References
Oseltamivir (Tamiflu)	Neuraminidase	Off-label use in birds; limited efficacy data	[29]
Zanamivir (Relenza)	Neuraminidase	Off-label use in birds; limited efficacy data	[30]
Peramivir	Neuraminidase	Off-label use in birds; limited efficacy data	[31]
Baloxavirmarboxil	Polymerase	Off-label use in birds; limited efficacy data	[32]
Favipiravir	Polymerase	Off-label use in birds; limited efficacy data	[33]
Amantadine	M2 ion channel	Resistance reported in avian influenza viruses.	[30]
Rimantadine	M2 ion channel	Resistance reported in avian influenza viruses.	[34]

Diagnosis

The diagnosis of H5N8 avian influenza is a complex process that combines laboratory testing, clinical assessment, and epidemiological research [35]. Initial suspicion is guided by clinical signs such as respiratory distress, lethargy, and decreased feed intake. However, laboratory tests such as RT-PCR for viral RNA detection and virus isolation from respiratory or tissue samples are necessary for confirmation. Pathological changes discovered during post-mortem examination help to further inform diagnosis. Antibodies are found by serological assays, which facilitate retroactive diagnosis [36]. Control measures are informed by epidemiological investigation, which clarifies routes of transmission. Effective management and timely reporting are ensured through collaboration among authorities, diagnostic laboratories, and veterinarians. Accurate diagnosis and surveillance are made possible by this all-encompassing approach, which is essential for reducing the impact of H5N8 on chicken populations.

Preventive Measures of H5N8 Avian Flu Virus

To stop and manage the spread of the H5N8 virus, also known as avian influenza or bird flu, strict biosecurity protocols are needed. Farm disinfection and access controls, early detection surveillance, prompt quarantine of contaminated flocks, culling when necessary, potential vaccination, and intensive education campaigns are a few of these. International cooperation is necessary for the exchange of information and coordinated responses. Research into improved diagnostics, vaccines, and control strategies is still essential to effectively lower the risks to the health of chickens and humans. Fig. (**2**) pictographically explains the preventive measures towards H5N8 Virus [37, 38].

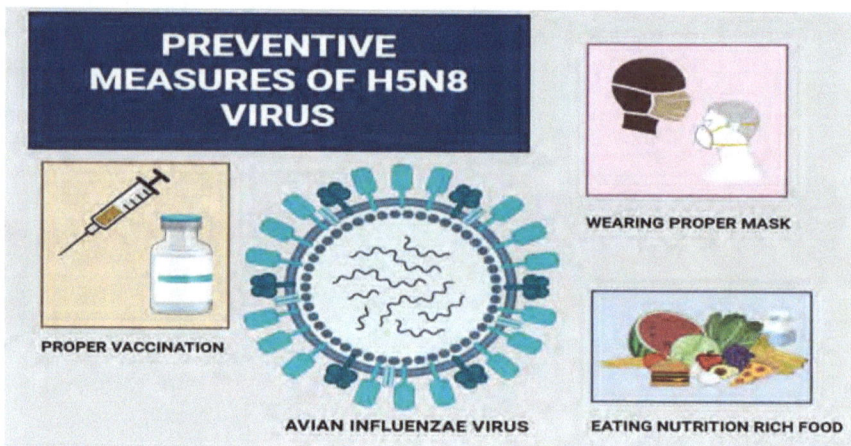

Fig. (2). Preventive measures of H5N8 Virus.

WHO Recommendations

The World Health Organization's Global Influenza Surveillance and Response System (GISRS) facilitates the vigilant monitoring of avian and other zoonotic influenza viruses [37]. WHO actively observes the human-animal interface, assesses associated risks, and coordinates responses to zoonotic influenza outbreaks and other public health crises in collaboration with the World Organisation for Animal Health (WOAH), the Food and Agriculture Organisation of the United Nations (FAO) and various partners. To scrutinize data on influenza viruses with pandemic potential generated by GISRS and animal health collaborators, WHO engages with experts from WHO Collaborating Centres, Essential Regulatory Laboratories, and other partners biannually [38]. The objective of these consultations is to determine the need for additional candidate vaccine viruses to enhance pandemic preparedness. To enhance both domestic and international preparedness and response, WHO evaluates risks, and formulates and refines strategies for surveillance, preparedness, and response to seasonal, zoonotic, and pandemic influenza [39]. The results of risk assessments and intervention recommendations are promptly communicated with member states. The WHO Pandemic Influenza Preparedness Framework serves as a global strategy for gearing up for the imminent influenza pandemic [40].

CONCLUSION

The highly pathogenic avian influenza A (H5N8) virus seriously threatens the world's poultry populations because of its rapid global spread and high pathogenicity. The present chapter thoroughly investigates the H5N8 virus, encompassing its composition, historical background, characteristics, frequency, case studies, therapeutic alternatives, diagnostic methodologies, and WHO guidelines. Birds are the main victims of the H5N8 virus, which mainly affects chicken populations and causes severe respiratory distress, decreased egg production, and high mortality rates. Its capacity to genetically reassort with other influenza subtypes adds to worries that it may develop into more virulent strains that can infect humans.

While human infections with H5N8 remain rare, the chapter highlights the importance of global surveillance, collaboration, and preparedness efforts to monitor and respond effectively to zoonotic influenza outbreaks. The World Health Organisation's global influenza surveillance and response system plays a crucial role in coordinating risk assessments, developing intervention strategies, and enhancing pandemic preparedness through global collaborations. Despite the availability of limited treatment options, such as antiviral medications like oseltamivir and zanamivir for off-label use in birds, the chapter emphasizes the significance of preventive measures, including stringent biosecurity protocols, surveillance, early detection, quarantine, and potential vaccination programs, to mitigate the impact of H5N8 on poultry health.

The case studies presented in this chapter underscore the widespread reach of H5N8 outbreaks across multiple countries, resulting in significant poultry deaths and economic losses. These incidents serve as a stark reminder of the virus's adaptability and the need for continuous research, vigilance, and international cooperation to develop improved diagnostics, vaccines, and control strategies. As the world grapples with the ongoing threat of emerging and re-emerging infectious diseases, this chapter provides a comprehensive resource for understanding the H5N8 avian influenza virus and serves as a call to action for concerted global efforts to safeguard animal and human health against potential pandemics.

AUTHORS CONTRIBUTION

Komal is responsible for writing and drafting this manuscript. Diksha, Brajesh Kumar Panda, Prabhjot Kaur, and Manish Kumar are responsible for the editing and Illustration of the manuscript. Dr. Amandeep Singh is responsible for the correspondence with the editor.

REFERENCES

[1]   Shi J, Zeng X, Cui P, Yan C, Chen H. Alarming situation of emerging H5 and H7 avian influenza and effective control strategies. Emerg Microbes Infect 2023; 12(1): 2155072.
        [http://dx.doi.org/10.1080/22221751.2022.2155072] [PMID: 36458831]

[2]   Rafique S, Rashid F, Mushtaq S, *et al.* Global review of the H5N8 avian influenza virus subtype. Front Microbiol 2023; 14: 1200681.
        [http://dx.doi.org/10.3389/fmicb.2023.1200681] [PMID: 37333639]

[3]   Yehia N, Salem HM, Mahmmod Y, *et al.* Common viral and bacterial avian respiratory infections: an updated review. Poult Sci 2023; 102(5): 102553.
        [http://dx.doi.org/10.1016/j.psj.2023.102553] [PMID: 36965253]

[4]   Si YJ, Park YR, Baek YG, *et al.* Pathogenesis and genetic characteristics of low pathogenic avian influenza H10 viruses isolated from migratory birds in South Korea during 2010–2019. Transbound Emerg Dis 2022; 69(5): 2588-99.
        [http://dx.doi.org/10.1111/tbed.14409] [PMID: 34863022]

[5]   Williams RAJ, Sánchez-Llatas CJ, Doménech A, *et al.* Emerging and novel viruses in passerine birds. Microorganisms 2023; 11(9): 2355.
        [http://dx.doi.org/10.3390/microorganisms11092355] [PMID: 37764199]

[6]   Xie R, Edwards KM, Wille M, *et al.* The episodic resurgence of highly pathogenic avian influenza H5 virus. Nature 2023; 622(7984): 810-7.
        [http://dx.doi.org/10.1038/s41586-023-06631-2] [PMID: 37853121]

[7]   Yang Q, Wang B, Lemey P, *et al.* Synchrony of bird migration with avian influenza global spread; implications for vulnerable bird orders. bioRxiv 2023; 2023.05.
        [http://dx.doi.org/10.1101/2023.05.22.541648]

[8]   Jiao C, Wang B, Chen P, Jiang Y, Liu J. Analysis of the conserved protective epitopes of hemagglutinin on influenza A viruses. Front Immunol 2023; 14: 1086297.
        [http://dx.doi.org/10.3389/fimmu.2023.1086297] [PMID: 36875062]

[9]   Djurdjević B, Polaček V, Pajić M, *et al.* Highly pathogenic avian influenza H5N8 outbreak in backyard chickens in Serbia. Animals (Basel) 2023; 13(4): 700.
        [http://dx.doi.org/10.3390/ani13040700] [PMID: 36830487]

[10]   Chauhan RP, Gordon ML. A systematic review of influenza A virus prevalence and transmission dynamics in backyard swine populations globally. Porcine Health Manag 2022; 8(1): 10.
        [http://dx.doi.org/10.1186/s40813-022-00251-4] [PMID: 35287744]

[11]   Yehia N, Naguib MM, Li R, *et al.* Multiple introductions of reassorted highly pathogenic avian influenza viruses (H5N8) clade 2.3.4.4b causing outbreaks in wild birds and poultry in Egypt. Infect Genet Evol 2018; 58: 56-65.
        [http://dx.doi.org/10.1016/j.meegid.2017.12.011] [PMID: 29248796]

[12]   Lycett SJ, Pohlmann A, Staubach C, *et al.* Genesis and spread of multiple reassortants during the 2016/2017 H5 avian influenza epidemic in Eurasia. Proc Natl Acad Sci USA 2020; 117(34): 20814-25.
        [http://dx.doi.org/10.1073/pnas.2001813117] [PMID: 32769208]

[13] Antigua KJC, Choi WS, Baek YH, Song MS. The emergence and decennary distribution of clade 2.3. 4.4 HPAI H5Nx. Microorganisms 2019; 7(6): 156.
[http://dx.doi.org/10.3390/microorganisms7060156] [PMID: 31146461]

[14] Salkeld D, Hopkins S, Hayman D. Emerging zoonotic and wildlife pathogens: disease ecology, epidemiology, and conservation. Oxford University Press 2023.
[http://dx.doi.org/10.1093/oso/9780198825920.001.0001]

[15] Zhang J, Li X, Wang X, *et al.* Genomic evolution, transmission dynamics, and pathogenicity of avian influenza A (H5N8) viruses emerging in China, 2020. Virus Evol 2021; 7(1): veab046.
[http://dx.doi.org/10.1093/ve/veab046] [PMID: 34141450]

[16] Adlhoch C, Fusaro A, Gonzales JL, *et al.* Avian influenza overview December 2022 - March 2023. EFSA J 2023; 21(3): e07917.
[PMID: 36949860]

[17] Banyard AC, Bennison A, Byrne AMP, *et al.* Detection and spread of high pathogenicity avian influenza virus H5N1 in the Antarctic Region. bioRxiv 2023; 2023.11.
[http://dx.doi.org/10.1101/2023.11.23.568045]

[18] Yamaguchi E, Hayama Y, Murato Y, Sawai K, Kondo S, Yamamoto T. A case-control study of the infection risk of H5N8 highly pathogenic avian influenza in Japan during the winter of 2020–2021. Res Vet Sci 2024; 168: 105149.
[http://dx.doi.org/10.1016/j.rvsc.2024.105149] [PMID: 38218062]

[19] Seo YR, Cho AY, Si YJ, *et al.* Evolution and spread of highly pathogenic avian influenza A(H5N1) clade 2.3.4.4b virus in wild birds, South Korea, 2022–2023. Emerg Infect Dis 2024; 30(2): 299-309.
[http://dx.doi.org/10.3201/eid3002.231274] [PMID: 38215495]

[20] El-Shall NA, Abd El Naby WSH, Hussein EGS, Yonis AE, Sedeik ME. Pathogenicity of H5N8 avian influenza virus in chickens and in duck breeds and the role of MX1 and IFN-α in infection outcome and transmission to contact birds. Comp Immunol Microbiol Infect Dis 2023; 100: 102039.
[http://dx.doi.org/10.1016/j.cimid.2023.102039] [PMID: 37591150]

[21] Yehia N, Rabie N, Adel A, *et al.* Differential replication characteristic of reassortant avian influenza A viruses H5N8 clade 2.3.4.4b in Madin-Darby canine kidney cell. Poult Sci 2023; 102(7): 102685.
[http://dx.doi.org/10.1016/j.psj.2023.102685] [PMID: 37267711]

[22] Niqueux É, Flodrops M, Allée C, *et al.* Evaluation of three hemagglutinin-based vaccines for the experimental control of a panzootic clade 2.3.4.4b A(H5N8) high pathogenicity avian influenza virus in mule ducks. Vaccine 2023; 41(1): 145-58.
[http://dx.doi.org/10.1016/j.vaccine.2022.11.012] [PMID: 36411134]

[23] Abolnik C, Ostmann E, Woods M, *et al.* Experimental infection of ostriches with H7N1 low pathogenic and H5N8 clade 2.3.4.4B highly pathogenic influenza A viruses. Vet Microbiol 2021; 263: 109251.
[http://dx.doi.org/10.1016/j.vetmic.2021.109251] [PMID: 34656859]

[24] Svyatchenko SV, Goncharova NI, Marchenko VY, *et al.* An influenza A(H5N8) virus isolated during an outbreak at a poultry farm in Russia in 2017 has an N294S substitution in the neuraminidase and shows reduced susceptibility to oseltamivir. Antiviral Res 2021; 191: 105079.
[http://dx.doi.org/10.1016/j.antiviral.2021.105079] [PMID: 33933515]

[25] Ibrahim M, Zakaria S, Bazid AHI, Kilany WH, Zain El-Abideen MA, Ali A. A single dose of inactivated oil-emulsion bivalent H5N8/H5N1 vaccine protects chickens against the lethal challenge of both highly pathogenic avian influenza viruses. Comp Immunol Microbiol Infect Dis 2021; 74: 101601.
[http://dx.doi.org/10.1016/j.cimid.2020.101601] [PMID: 33307456]

[26] Hassan KE, King J, El-Kady M, *et al.* Novel reassortant highly pathogenic avian influenza A (H5N2) virus in broiler chickens, Egypt. Emerg Infect Dis 2020; 26(1): 129-33.

[http://dx.doi.org/10.3201/eid2601.190570] [PMID: 31855539]

[27]   Shehata AA, Sedeik ME, Elbestawy AR, *et al.* Co-infections, genetic, and antigenic relatedness of avian influenza H5N8 and H5N1 viruses in domestic and wild birds in Egypt. Poult Sci 2019; 98(6): 2371-9.
[http://dx.doi.org/10.3382/ps/pez011] [PMID: 30668795]

[28]   Akter S, Alhatlani BY, Abdallah EM, *et al.* Exploring cinnamoyl-substituted mannopyranosides: synthesis, evaluation of antimicrobial properties, and molecular docking studies targeting h5n1 influenza a virus. Molecules 2023; 28(24): 8001.
[http://dx.doi.org/10.3390/molecules28248001] [PMID: 38138491]

[29]   Murray J, Martin DE, Sancilio FD, Tripp RA. Antiviral activity of probenecid and oseltamivir on influenza virus replication. Viruses 2023; 15(12): 2366.
[http://dx.doi.org/10.3390/v15122366] [PMID: 38140606]

[30]   Jones JC, Yen HL, Adams P, *et al.* Influenza antivirals and their role in pandemic preparedness. Antiviral Res 2023; 210: 105499.
[http://dx.doi.org/10.1016/j.antiviral.2022.105499] [PMID: 36567025]

[31]   Alasiri A, Soltane R, Hegazy A, *et al.* Vaccination and antiviral treatment against Avian influenza H5Nx viruses: a harbinger of virus control or evolution. Vaccines (Basel) 2023; 11(11): 1628.
[http://dx.doi.org/10.3390/vaccines11111628] [PMID: 38005960]

[32]   Guan W, Qu R, Shen L. *et al.* Baloxavir marboxil use for critical human infection of avian influenza A H5N6 virus. Med, 2024. 5(1): p. 32-41. e5.
[http://dx.doi.org/10.1016/j.medj.2023.11.001]

[33]   Yash S, Sarika K, Laxmikant B. Favipiravir: an effective rna polymerase modulating anti-influenza drug. Biosci Biotechnol Res Asia 2023; 20(2): 465-75.
[http://dx.doi.org/10.13005/bbra/3102]

[34]   Chakraborty S, Chauhan A. Anti-influenza agents. viral infections and antiviral therapies. Elsevier 2023; pp. 211-39.
[http://dx.doi.org/10.1016/B978-0-323-91814-5.00006-4]

[35]   Tran TD, Kasemsuwan S, Sukmak M, *et al.* Field and laboratory investigation of highly pathogenic avian influenza H5N6 and H5N8 in Quang Ninh province, Vietnam, 2020 to 2021. J Vet Sci 2024; 25(2): e20.
[http://dx.doi.org/10.4142/jvs.23184] [PMID: 38568822]

[36]   Maartens LH, Frizzo da Silva L, Dawson S, Love N, Erasmus BJ. The efficacy of an inactivated avian influenza H5N1 vaccine against an African strain of HPAI H5N8 (clade 2.3.4.4 B). Avian Pathol 2023; 52(3): 176-84.
[http://dx.doi.org/10.1080/03079457.2023.2181145] [PMID: 37079321]

[37]   Adlhoch C, Fusaro A, Gonzales JL, *et al.* Avian influenza overview December 2020 - February 2021. EFSA J 2021; 19(3): e06497.
[PMID: 33717356]

[38]   Sands P, Winters J. Countering the pandemic threat through global coordination on vaccines: the influenza imperative. National Academies of Sciences, Engineering, and Medicine 2021.

[39]   Organization WH. Report of the annual meeting to review the progress of the implementation of the pandemic influenza preparedness (PIP) partnership contribution (PC) funds in the WHO South-East Asia Region [hybrid] 18–19 October 2022, New Delhi, India. 2023, World Health Organization. Regional Office for South-East Asia.

[40]   Keränen LB. Preparing for pandemic: securitizing rhetoric in us national influenza response plans, 1978-2017. Rhetoric of Health & Medicine, 2023. 6(4).

Ebola in the Democratic Republic of Congo: A Guide to Prevention, Treatment, and WHO Recommendations

Animesh Ranjan[1], Rakesh Chawla[2], Neeraj Patil[1], Diksha[3], Brajesh Kumar Panda[3], Dhritisri Dutta[4], Naresh Kumar Ranrga[5] and Amandeep Singh[6,*]

[1] *Department of Regulatory Affairs, ISF College of Pharmacy, Moga, Punjab-142001, India*

[2] *Department of Pharma Chemistry, University Institute of Pharmacy, Baba Farid University of Health Sciences, Faridkot, Punjab-151203, India*

[3] *Department of Quality Assurance, ISF College of Pharmacy, Moga, Punjab-142001, India*

[4] *Department of Pharmacy Practice, ISF College of Pharmacy, Moga, Punjab-142001, India*

[5] *Department of Pharmaceutical Chemistry, ISF College of Pharmacy, Moga, Punjab-142001, India*

[6] *Department of Pharmaceutics, ISF College of Pharmacy, Moga, Punjab-142001, India*

Abstract: On December 16, 2021, the outbreak of Ebola Virus Disease (EVD) in the Beni Health Zone, North Kivu Province, Democratic Republic of the Congo, was officially declared over. This marked the end of the outbreak, which began on October 8, 2021. So far 11 outbreaks have been recorded, of which two survived and nine died. This chapter discusses various factors such as epidemiological features, modes of transmission, clinical symptoms, infection, prevalence, surveillance strategies, prevention strategies, treatment options, and WHO recommendations summary of the epidemic. Most cases involve kids under the age of five, highlighting their vulnerability. Strong preventive measures, such as quarantine, contact management, safe burials and vaccination campaigns brought an end to the outbreak. The Ebola virus characteristics, exposure time, mortality and symptoms are discussed, and the severity and complications are emphasized with implications for public health. Virus physiology includes immune evasion mechanisms, regulation of cytokine/chemokine networks, and inhibition of type I independent responses. The frequency of Ebola is analysed, with outbreaks occurring most frequently in countries in Central and West Africa. Spread is affected by animal vectors, modes of transmission, and social influences. Vaccine use and advances in treatment, surveillance strategies, prevention programs and treatment are all discussed. WHO guidelines strongly emphasize comprehensive care for EVD victims, preparedness in health facilities, community involvement, and infection control measures. Preventing an Ebola outbreak effectively

---

* **Corresponding author Amandeep Singh:** Department of Pharmaceutics, ISF College of Pharmacy, Moga, Punjab-142001, India; E-mail: ad4singh@gmail.com

minimizing its impact on global health requires improved public health policy, international cooperation, and ongoing research.

Keywords: Case fatality rate, Democratic republic of congo, Ebola virus disease, Zoonotic transmission, Outbreak.

INTRODUCTION

On December 16, 2021, the Democratic Republic of the Congo's Ministry of Health officially declared the conclusion of the Ebola virus disease (EVD) outbreak in Beni Health Zone, North Kivu Province, by WHO guidelines, 42 days after the last confirmed case tested negative for the second time [1, 2]. Between October 8 and December 16, a total of 11 cases were reported in Beni HZ, including eight confirmed and three probable cases, resulting in nine deaths and two survivors. The overall case fatality ratio (CFR) stands at 82% among total cases and 75% among confirmed cases [3, 4]. The outbreak, declared on October 8, began with a 3-year-old boy exhibiting symptoms such as weakness, loss of appetite, abdominal pain, breathing difficulties, and gastrointestinal issues [5]. The emergence of Ebola outbreaks transcends the realm of public health, triggering a cascade of profound social, economic, and psychological ramifications within affected communities. These consequences often manifest as heightened fear, social stigma, and disruptions to both healthcare infrastructure and the daily routines of individuals [6]. Ebola, a severe illness from the Ebola virus, lurks in wild animals like fruit bats. Human outbreaks, concentrated in Central and West Africa, arise from contact with infected animals. This highly contagious virus spreads through bodily fluids, and healthcare hygiene is crucial. Symptoms like fever and bleeding appear after 2-21 days. Beyond the health crisis, Ebola outbreaks disrupt societies and inflict fear [1].

CHARACTERISTICS

Transmission

Natural Reservoir: The Ebola virus is hypothesized to have a natural reservoir in specific animal species, such as fruit bats. Zoonotic transmission events, marked by the initial transfer of the virus from these animal reservoirs to humans, are believed to be the origin of Ebola virus outbreaks. These transmission events are most likely to occur during activities that involve the handling or consumption of infected animals [7, 8]. Ebola virus infection presents with a variety of clinical manifestations, including elevated body temperature, intense cephalalgia, myalgia, profound asthenia, diarrhoea, emesis, stomachache, and uncontrolled haemorrhage or ecchymosis [9, 10]. Fatality Rate (CFR): Ebola outbreaks exhibit a high case fatality rate, varying between outbreaks but often reaching alarming levels. The CFR can be influenced by factors such as healthcare infrastructure, early detection, and access to medical care. Incubation Period: Ebola exhibits an incubation period ranging from 2 to 21 days. Notably, during this interval, infected individuals may remain asymptomatic; however, they are still capable of transmitting the virus to others [11]. Nosocomial Spread: Geographic Distribution: Documented Ebola outbreaks have been concentrated in Central and West Africa, with the identification of distinct viral strains. The geographical spread of these outbreaks exhibits variability, ranging from isolated occurrences in rural areas to episodes affecting densely populated urban centres [12]. Community Impact: The emergence of Ebola outbreaks transcends the realm of public health, triggering a cascade of profound social, economic, and psychological ramifications within affected communities. These consequences often manifest as heightened fear, social stigma, and disruptions to both healthcare infrastructure and the daily routines of individuals.

Outbreak Control Measures: Control measures during Ebola outbreaks include case isolation, contact tracing, safe burials, community engagement, and the implementation of infection prevention and control measures in healthcare settings [13].Vaccination Efforts: In recent years, efforts to control Ebola outbreaks have included the deployment of vaccines, such as rVSV-ZEBOV-GP, as a preventive measure for individuals at risk of exposure [14].

Features of Ebola Virus: Structure, Transmission and Clinical Manifestation

Ebola, a thread-like virus with a protective outer shell, belongs to a family of viruses known for causing severe illness. This unique structure and other characteristics of Ebola play a big role in how it makes people sick [15]. Examining these features is crucial for understanding the virus's biology, transmission dynamics, and the development of effective countermeasures. The Ebola virus carries its instructions in a single, coiled-up strand of RNA, kind of like a recipe. This genetic material is around 19,000 to 30,000 letters long and contains the code for building seven different parts, or proteins, that the virus needs to function [16]. The Ebola virus is like a tiny machine with seven different parts, each with a specific function. One particularly important part is the surface glycoprotein (GP). This protein acts like a key, allowing the virus to enter human cells. Because it is so crucial for infection, the body's immune system also tries hard to target and inactivate this protein [17]. There are five different types of Ebola virus: Zaire, Sudan, Tai Forest, Bundibugyo, and Reston [18]. Different types (species) of Ebola virus can be found in different areas of the world, and some cause more severe illness than others. For example, the Zaire species is known to be particularly deadly [19], while the Reston species, although pathogenic to non-human primates, has not caused significant disease in humans [20]. The natural reservoir for the Ebola virus is believed to be fruit bats [21], particularly those of the Pteropodidae family. Transmission to humans typically occurs through the handling or consumption of infected animals, such as bats or primates. This zoonotic transmission is a key factor in the initiation of Ebola virus outbreaks. Human-to-human transmission of the Ebola virus is a defining feature of its epidemiology. This occurs through direct contact with the blood, secretions, organs, or other bodily fluids of infected individuals [7]. Ebola outbreaks are especially risky in hospitals and clinics, where the virus can easily spread from person to person. This highlights the importance of strict hygiene protocols for healthcare workers. People infected with Ebola experience a range of severe symptoms. These can include fever, headaches so bad they're hard to bear, muscle aches, extreme tiredness, diarrhea, vomiting, stomach pain, and bleeding or bruising that appears for no reason [22]. The severity of symptoms can vary, with some individuals remaining asymptomatic carriers of the virus. The incubation period for Ebola virus infection ranges from 2 to 21 days [23]. During this period, People can spread the virus before showing symptoms, making it harder to control outbreaks [23]. This poses challenges for early detection and containment efforts during outbreaks. One of the most alarming features of Ebola virus outbreaks is the high case fatality rate (CFR), which can range from 25% to 90%, depending on the virus strain and the availability of medical care [24]. This underscores the urgency of effective treatments and supportive care during outbreaks. The Ebola virus has evolved mechanisms to evade the host's immune response, contributing to its ability to establish infection and cause severe diseases. Paradoxically, the severity of Ebola virus disease is associated with a dysregulated immune response, leading to immunosuppression [25]. In recent years, efforts to combat Ebola virus outbreaks have included the deployment of vaccines, such as rVSV-ZEBOV-GP, as preventive measures for individuals at risk of exposure [26]. These vaccines have shown promise in clinical trials, offering hope for improved control and prevention strategies in the future. The Ebola virus exhibits a complex array of features that contribute to its pathogenicity and impact on human health. From its genetic structure and surface glycoprotein to its zoonotic transmission and severe clinical manifestations, understanding these features is crucial for developing effective diagnostic tools, vaccines, and treatments to combat Ebola virus infections and mitigate the impact of outbreaks on global public health. health. Below, Table **1** provides the symptomology of Ebola Virus [23-25].

Table 1. Signs and symptoms of the ebola virus.

Initial Symptoms	Fever, Myalgia, Malaise, Sore Throat
Gastrointestinal symptom	Nausea, Vomiting, Diarrhea, Dehydration, Abdominal pain, GI bleeding

(Table 1) cont.....

Initial Symptoms	Fever, Myalgia, Malaise, Sore Throat
Hemorrhagic symptom	Bruises, Petechia
Ophthalmic symptom	Uveitis
Neurological symptom	Delirium, confusion, coma
Shock or organ failure	Hypotension, Tachycardia, and Failure of organs such as the kidney, liver, and adrenal glands.

Pathogenesis

Ebolaviruses are 19 kb negative-strand RNA viruses from the Filoviridae family. The virus is filamentous and pleomorphic, with an average unit length of 1200 nm [26]. The Ebola virus genome is like a code with seven instructions, each in a specific order. These instructions tell the virus how to make the proteins it needs (nucleoprotein, VP35, VP40, glycoprotein, VP30, VP24, and polymerase) and end with a special closing section. EBOV replicates in antigen-presenting cells, including macrophages and dendritic cells (DCs). However, the virus can infect a wide range of cell types, including endothelium and epithelial cells, fibroblasts, hepatocytes, macrophages, monocytes, DCs, Kupffer cells, and cells of adrenal gland tissue. These infections may eventually lead to an increase in viremia. The signs and symptoms of Ebola Virus Disease (EVD), like the immune system's struggles and bleeding problems, seem to be caused by the Ebola virus (EBOV) damaging and killing cells in the body. When the Ebola virus (EBOV) infects someone, it disrupts their immune system in several ways. For instance, it can prevent the body from producing a key antiviral weapon called interferon, mess up the immune system's signalling system, and weaken certain immune cells that normally fight infection. Our bodies have a natural defense system called interferons (IFNs) that help fight viruses. There are different types of IFNs, and some are particularly good at stopping infections early on. Unfortunately, the Ebola virus (EBOV) can block these beneficial interferons, making it harder for the body to fight back. The Ebola virus (EBOV) has several tricks to weaken the body's defences. It can stop infected immune cells from making interferons (IFNs) on their own, and it can also prevent other signals from triggering the production of IFNs. EBOV has two proteins involved in this process: VP35 messes up an important pathway for making a specific type of IFN (IFN-β), and VP24 throws a wrench into how all IFNs work by interfering with their signalling system. This inhibits the transcription of antiviral genes [28]. Ebola throws a curveball at our immune system, making it harder to fight back. Even though the body tries to cook up special defences against Ebola, the virus often comes out on top in this battle. Fig. (1) provides an overview on the pathogenesis of Ebola Virus [27-29]. This idea of a constant struggle between the body and the virus might also be key to understanding how vaccines protect us from Ebola. Once outside the window for a vaccine-induced mounting of a humoral response, a vaccinated individual is thought to be protected [29].

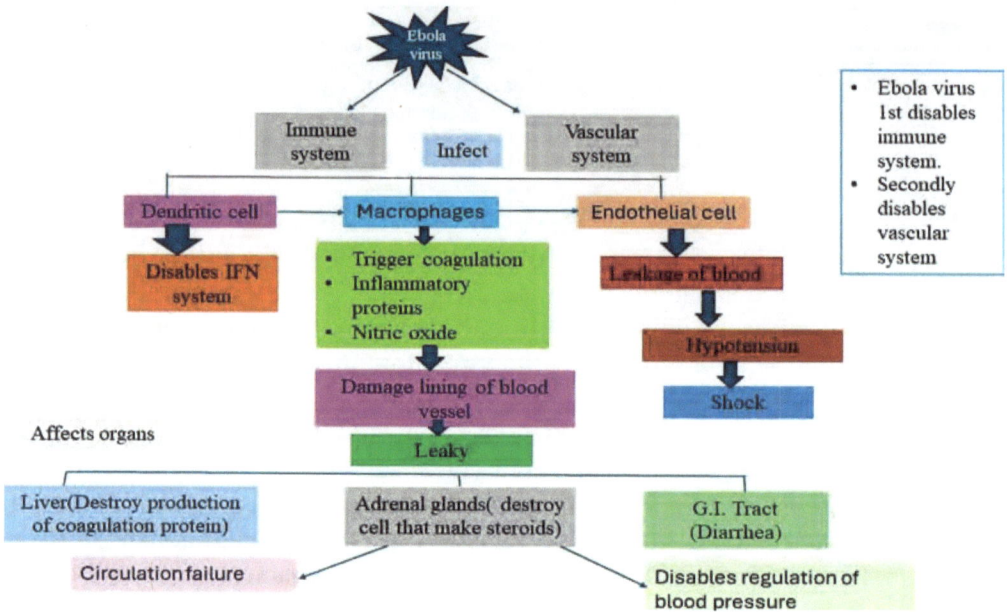

Fig. (1). Pathogenesis of ebola virus [27 - 29].

Prevalence

The prevalence of the Ebola virus, a highly pathogenic and often fatal virus, has been a recurring concern, particularly in sub-Saharan Africa where outbreaks have occurred sporadically since the virus's discovery in 1976 [30]. To understand how much Ebola affects people, we need to look at where it shows up, how widespread it is in those areas, and how it harms communities. It is important to note that Ebola outbreaks have happened mainly in countries located in Central and West Africa. Ebola first showed up in 1976, hitting what are now two separate countries: the Democratic Republic of Congo and South Sudan [31]. Since then, outbreaks have been documented in various countries, including Sudan, Uganda, Gabon, the Republic of Congo, Ivory Coast, and Guinea. The name "Ebola" actually comes from the Ebola River in the Democratic Republic of Congo (DRC). This river is significant because the very first outbreak of the virus ever identified occurred near its banks [32]. The prevalence of Ebola is closely tied to the presence of the virus in its natural reservoirs, which are believed to be fruit bats, particularly those of the Pteropodidae family. These bats may carry the virus asymptomatically and can transmit it to other animals or humans through direct or indirect contact. One of the distinctive features of Ebola virus prevalence is its episodic and unpredictable nature [33]. Outbreaks do not follow a regular pattern, and their occurrence can be influenced by various factors, including ecological, epidemiological, and human behavioral factors. For instance, factors such as deforestation, climate change, and increased human interactions with wildlife may contribute to the emergence of the virus [34, 35]. Ebola's impact is not limited to just how often it appears. The severity of the illness it causes also plays a big role. This is measured by the case fatality rate (CFR), which basically means what percentage of people infected with Ebola die. It is important to note that this CFR can vary depending on a few things. The specific strain of the virus itself can make a difference, as can access to proper medical care and how quickly public health officials can react to an outbreak [36]. The Zaire Ebola virus species, in particular, has been associated with high CFRs, reaching up to 90% in some instances [37]. Transmission dynamics play a crucial role in the prevalence of Ebola. Ebola spreads from person to person when someone touches the blood, vomit, sweat, or other bodily fluids of an infected person [38]. Nosocomial transmission, or transmission within healthcare settings, has been a significant factor in some outbreaks, emphasizing the importance of infection prevention and control measures. While the majority of Ebola outbreaks have been confined to rural areas, urban outbreaks pose unique challenges due to increased population density and mobility. Urban settings can facilitate rapid virus spread, making containment efforts more complex [39]. The World Health Organization (WHO) and other international health organizations are like firefighters for Ebola outbreaks. They constantly watch for them and jump in to help when they happen. Surveillance systems are in place to detect and confirm cases promptly, enabling a swift response to contain the virus's spread. The deployment of diagnostic tests, such as reverse transcription-polymerase chain reaction (RT-PCR), has improved the accuracy and speed of case identification [40]. Prevalence is not only about the number of cases but also about the societal impact of the virus. Ebola outbreaks have profound social, economic, and psychological consequences on affected communities. Fear, stigma, and disruptions to healthcare and daily life are common outcomes, exacerbating the challenges of controlling the virus [41]. Efforts to combat the prevalence of Ebola include the development and deployment of vaccines. The rVSV-ZEBOV-GP vaccine has shown efficacy in clinical trials, offering a preventive measure for individuals at risk of exposure. Vaccination campaigns have been initiated in response to outbreaks to create a ring of immunity around confirmed cases and contacts [42]. The global community recognizes the need for a comprehensive and collaborative approach to address the prevalence of the Ebola virus. This includes strengthening healthcare systems, improving surveillance and response capabilities, and engaging communities in preventive measures. International partnerships and research efforts contribute to developing better diagnostics, treatments, and vaccines to enhance our ability to control and prevent Ebola outbreaks. In conclusion, the prevalence of the Ebola virus is a dynamic and complex phenomenon shaped by ecological, epidemiological, and human factors. Understanding and addressing the virus's prevalence require ongoing research, international collaboration, and a commitment to strengthening public health systems to effectively respond to outbreaks and mitigate the impact on affected communities.

SURVEILLANCE

Prevention Against EBOD

Ebola has two main ways of spreading. People can get it from infected animals, especially fruit bats, or through close contact with the bodily fluids of someone who's sick. This highlights the risk from both the animal world and from infected people. To stop the spread, health officials identify and isolate sick people, track their contacts, and educate the public about the disease [41]. To protect healthcare workers from Ebola, experienced organizations like the WHO recommend specific precautions. These include standard hygiene practices, using protective gear that fully covers the body (like Tyvek suits), and wearing specialized masks that filter air (powered air-purifying respirators or PAPRs). If PAPRs are not available, N95 masks can be used, although they offer less protection. Four vaccinations have been approved by different regulatory organizations. Several vaccines protect against Ebola by introducing a harmless copy of the Ebola virus's surface protein (GP) into the body. This triggers the immune system to learn how to fight the real virus. There are different approaches to delivering this GP protein: Ervebo uses a modified vesicular stomatitis virus, while Zabdeno/Mvabea and Ad5-EBOV use adenoviruses. GamEvac-Combi combines both methods for potentially stronger immunity. Only Zabdeno/Mvabea, which contains Mvabea, targets many species of the Ebolavirus genus among the already licensed vaccines. Ervebo (rVSV-EBOV) is a live-attenuated, replication-competent vaccine licensed by the FDA and the European Medicines Agency (EMA) that is given as a single dose. It is a genetically engineered form of the VSV, an animal virus that contains EBOV's GP. It has demonstrated significant immunogenicity and durability, with EBOV GP-specific antibodies surviving for up to two years after vaccination. Furthermore, while there are a few trials examining its safety in infants, pregnant and breastfeeding women, the WHO supports its use in active EBV epidemic areas.

Treatment Modalities

The fight against Ebola involves exploring new treatment options. Promising medications like GP and PI inhibitors are undergoing initial tests with positive results. While existing drugs have not been effective beyond lab settings, advancements in AI and machine learning offer hope. These technologies can analyse vast amounts of chemical data to identify potential new treatments for Ebola [40]. Machine learning (ML) is the process of analysing data, drawing conclusions from it, and forecasting or judging the future state of any newly created dataset. Therefore, computers are taught how to complete tasks using massive volumes of data and algorithms rather than programmers manually developing software routines with a specific set of instructions to accomplish a given task. Two popular machine learning techniques are supervised and unsupervised learning, which use labelled data for training. Deep neural networks are used in specific applications to integrate and evaluate genetic, epidemiological, and meteorological data, and natural language processing is used to extract insights from unstructured text-based reports [40]. Host factors that are involved in immune response and viral activities have gained interest as potential targets for therapy recently. Amiodarone was tried in Sierra Leone but was eventually pulled out due to conflicting results in animal models, despite being demonstrated to prevent viral membrane fusion *in vitro*. In order to reduce drug dosage and toxicity and avoid resistance, combination therapy, which comprises FDA-approved drugs (toremifene-clarithromycin-posaconazole and toremifene-mefloquine-posaconazole), has been developed. *In vitro* studies have demonstrated the ability of these suggested combinations to block different stages of viral entrance and reproduction. Scientists are excited about a new type of drug called AAK1 inhibitors to fight viruses like Ebola. These drugs seem to work by blocking a critical pathway that viruses use to enter human cells. One example, a combination of Sunitinib and Erlotinib, has shown promise against Ebola in lab studies.

WHO Recommendations

Protecting ourselves from diseases that can jump from wild animals to humans is important. This is especially true for viruses carried by fruit bats, monkeys, and apes. To minimize this risk, anyone handling these animals should always wear gloves and suitable protective clothing. This creates a barrier that helps prevent germs from spreading between humans and wild animals. Prior to consumption, thorough cooking of animal products such as blood and meat is imperative. To curb human-to-human transmission, particularly from close contact with individuals displaying Ebola symptoms and their bodily fluids, it is essential to wear suitable personal 181N390604TM001H protective equipment. Rigorous handwashing is mandatory after interacting with patients in healthcare settings and after any contact with bodily fluids. Even after recovering from Ebola, the virus might linger in some body fluids for a while. To address this, the World

Health Organization (WHO) recommends a comprehensive care program for survivors. This program includes complete medical care, mental health support, and repeated testing to ensure the virus is cleared from the body (shown by two negative tests in a row). Importantly, the WHO does not recommend isolating survivors who have already tested negative for Ebola [39]. To effectively fight Ebola, healthcare workers need ongoing training on how to spot cases early, isolate patients safely, and provide proper treatment. This training emphasizes safe and respectful burial practices that follow infection control protocols. Having enough personal protective equipment (PPE) and infection prevention supplies is also vital. This gear protects healthcare workers while they care for sick patients and properly clean contaminated areas [40, 41]. Health facility assessments, including a "Scorecard," should be conducted to evaluate adherence to IPC measures in preparation for handling Ebola patients, encompassing aspects such as water, sanitation, hygiene (WASH), waste management, PPE supplies, and triage/screening capacity [42]. Engagement with communities is vital to reinforce safe and dignified burial practices, fostering a collaborative effort to prevent the spread of Ebola.

ROLE OF MULTI-AGENCIES IN THE MANAGEMENT OF VIRAL DISEASES

The One Health concept acknowledges the interdependence of environmental, animal, and human health through a holistic and integrated method. Instead of concentrating only on measures pertaining to human health, it encourages cross-sectoral collaboration to address the underlying causes of zoonotic illnesses like Ebola.

Public Health Agencies

World Health Organization (WHO)

In organizing global initiatives for disease surveillance, epidemic investigation, emergency response, and capacity building, WHO is a major player. In order to contain outbreaks, they work with governments and partners to develop procedures for diagnosis and treatment, as well as to provide technical instructions [43].

Centres for Disease Control and Prevention (CDC)

The CDC assists with outbreak detection, offers epidemiological guidance, and creates response plans. They frequently deploy field teams to help with outbreak management during Ebola epidemics, which includes monitoring cases, establishing isolation units, and educating nearby healthcare professionals [44].

Animal Health Agencies

Food and Agriculture Organization (FAO)

The FAO plays a role by keeping an eye on animal health, especially in wildlife populations that serve as breeding grounds for zoonotic viruses like Ebola. By providing veterinarian resources and putting up early warning systems, they help restrict the transmission of animal diseases to people [45].

World Organisation for Animal Health (OIE)

OIE helps governments in managing diseases in livestock and animals that potentially endanger human health, with a focus on animal disease surveillance. It is crucial to recognize and control possible animal carriers of the Ebola virus, such as fruit bats [46].

National Governments

To establish a comprehensive strategy for epidemic management, governments collaborate across sectors, supervising agencies involved in border security, agriculture, healthcare, and the environment. Working with international partners, they mobilise resources, enforce quarantines, disseminate public health information, and guarantee that safety protocols are followed.

Environmental and Wildlife Agencies

United Nations Environment Programme (UNEP)

UNEP studies the relationship between human encroachment into wildlife habitats, deforestation, biodiversity loss, and other ecological factors and the spread of illnesses like Ebola. It is their responsibility to suggest environmental laws that lessen the possibility of zoonotic spillovers [47].

THE ROLE OF "ONE HEALTH" STRATEGIES IN MANAGING VIRAL DISEASES

The One Health strategy acknowledges the relationship between animal, environmental, and human health through an integrated, interdisciplinary approach. In order to better prevent, identify, and treat viral diseases—particularly those that are zoonotic, or able to transmit between people and animals—it encourages cooperation between various sectors. The interdependence of human, animal, and environmental health has been highlighted by viral infections such as COVID-19, Zika, Ebola, and influenza, underscoring the growing relevance of the One Health concept.

Surveillance and Early Detection

Monitoring human, animal, and environmental health is emphasised by One Health in order to identify newly developing viral infections early on. Potential viral dangers like Ebola and Avian Influenza can be detected before they infect humans by monitoring domestic animals, livestock, and wildlife. Tracking environmental variables like deforestation and climate change aids in the prediction of viral transmission. Furthermore, coordinating efforts between the agricultural and health sectors to integrate veterinary and human health data improves the early identification of zoonotic diseases.

Coordinated Response

One Health brings together professionals in health, animal welfare, and the environment to promote multi-sectoral cooperation during viral epidemics. As demonstrated by the Ebola epidemics, this cooperation aids in the containment of viruses in both animal and human populations. To stem the spread of zoonotic viruses such as MERS or Nipah, rapid reaction teams made up of veterinarians, healthcare professionals, and environmental specialists track down the diseases. Sharing resources—labs, staff, and vaccinations—improves epidemic control by accelerating diagnosis, guaranteeing effective treatment, and distributing immunizations.

Prevention and Risk Reduction

One Health manages animal reservoirs by implementing strategies including immunising cattle and controlling the trade in wildlife in order to stop viral spillovers. In order to lessen human-wildlife interactions—which are frequently the source of infections like Ebola and Hantavirus—it also places a strong emphasis on biodiversity protection and sustainable land use. One Health also encourages community education to increase knowledge of the links between human, animal, and environmental health. Campaigns for public health work to deter dangerous behaviours, such as eating bushmeat, which lowers the likelihood of zoonotic disease epidemics.

Research and Development of Vaccines and Treatments

Especially for zoonotic viruses, One Health fosters the development of vaccines and antivirals against all species. Experts in veterinary and human health may work together more quickly thanks to shared research platforms, which help develop vaccines that target both animal and human reservoirs, like in the case of coronavirus research. This strategy also supports vaccinations with two purposes, such as the Hendra virus vaccine, which was first created for horses but is also successful in stopping the virus from spreading to people. This illustrates the advantages of immunising both groups at the same time [48, 49].

CONCLUSION

The Ebola virus disease (EVD) remains a significant public health threat, especially in Central and West Africa, where outbreaks have occurred sporadically since its discovery in 1976. The high case fatality rates associated with EVD, combined with its ability to spread through human-to-human transmission, underscore the urgency of developing effective countermeasures.

Understanding the unique features of the Ebola virus, including its structure, pathogenesis, and transmission dynamics, is crucial for advancing diagnostics, treatments, and prevention strategies. While progress has been made in areas such as vaccine development and deployment, much work remains to be done. Controlling and preventing Ebola outbreaks requires a multifaceted approach that encompasses strengthening healthcare systems, improving surveillance and response capabilities, and engaging communities in preventive measures. International collaboration and ongoing research efforts are vital to address the challenges posed by the Ebola virus and mitigate its impact on global health.

Ultimately, the successful management of Ebola outbreaks hinges on a comprehensive and coordinated response from the global health community. By leveraging scientific advancements, fostering international partnerships, and prioritizing public health preparedness, we can enhance our ability to combat this formidable virus and protect vulnerable populations from its devastating effects.

AUTHOR CONTRIBUTION

Animesh, Neeraj Patil, Dhritishri Dutta, and Diksha are responsible for the drafting and editing of the Book Chapter. Dr. N.K. Rangra is responsible for the correspondence with the editor.

REFERENCES

[1]   Sah R, Mohanty A, Mehta V, Satapathy P, Padhi BK, Rodriguez-Morales AJ. The ebola resurgence in democratic republic of congo. Ann Med Surg (Lond) 2022; 82: 104616.
       [http://dx.doi.org/10.1016/j.amsu.2022.104616] [PMID: 36124213]

[2]   Prevention, C.f.D.C.A. History of Ebola Disease Outbreaks. 15.03.2024]; Available from: https://www.cdc.gov/vhf/ebola/history/chronology.html

[3]   Vossler H, Akilimali P, Pan Y, KhudaBukhsh WR, Kenah E, Rempała GA. Analysis of individual-level data from 2018–2020 Ebola outbreak in Democratic Republic of the Congo. Sci Rep 2022; 12(1): 5534.
       [http://dx.doi.org/10.1038/s41598-022-09564-4] [PMID: 35365724]

[4]   Organization, W.H. Ebola virus disease –Democratic Republic of the Congo. 15.03.2024]; Available

from: https://www.who.int/emergencies/disease-outbreak-news/item/2022-DON411

[5]   Sun J, Uwishema O, Kassem H, *et al.* Ebola virus outbreak returns to the Democratic Republic of Congo: An urgent rising concern. Ann Med Surg (Lond) 2022; 79: 103958.
[http://dx.doi.org/10.1016/j.amsu.2022.103958] [PMID: 35757313]

[6]   Organisation, W.H. Ebola virus disease – Democratic Republic of the Congo. 15.03.2024]; Available from: https://www.who.int/emergencies/disease-outbreak-news/item/2021-DON351

[7]   Rewar S, Mirdha D. Transmission of ebola virus disease: an overview. Ann Glob Health 2015; 80(6): 444-51.
[http://dx.doi.org/10.1016/j.aogh.2015.02.005] [PMID: 25960093]

[8]   Gebretadik F, Seifu M, Gelaw B. Review on Ebola virus disease: its outbreak and current status. 2015.

[9]   Osterholm MT, Moore KA, Kelley NS. *et al.* Transmission of Ebola viruses: what we know and what we do not know. MBio, 2015. 6(2): p. 10.1128/mbio. 00137-15.
[http://dx.doi.org/10.1128/mBio.00137-15]

[10]   Raza A, Rahman MA. Ebola virus disease prevention and control. Int J 2020; 3(1): 419.

[11]   America, I.D.s.O. Ebola Facts. 16.03.2024]; Available from: https://www.idsociety.org/public-health/ebola/ebola-resources/ebola-facts

[12]   Aitken C, Jeffries DJ. Nosocomial spread of viral disease. Clin Microbiol Rev 2001; 14(3): 528-46.
[http://dx.doi.org/10.1128/CMR.14.3.528-546.2001] [PMID: 11432812]

[13]   Coltart CEM, Lindsey B, Ghinai I, Johnson AM, Heymann DL. The Ebola outbreak, 2013–2016: old lessons for new epidemics. Philos Trans R Soc Lond B Biol Sci 2017; 372(1721): 20160297.
[http://dx.doi.org/10.1098/rstb.2016.0297] [PMID: 28396469]

[14]   Thippeswamy NB. Immunological mechanisms associated with clinical features of Ebola virus disease and its control and prevention.Pandemic Outbreaks in the 21st Century. Elsevier 2021; pp. 159-83.
[http://dx.doi.org/10.1016/B978-0-323-85662-1.00001-X]

[15]   Brown, K.S., A. Silaghi, and H. Feldmann, Ebolavirus, in Encyclopedia of Virology (Third Edition), B.W.J. Mahy and M.H.V. Van Regenmortel, Editors. 2008, Academic Press: Oxford. p. 57-65.

[16]   Jain S, Martynova E, Rizvanov A, Khaiboullina S, Baranwal M. Structural and functional aspects of ebola virus proteins. Pathogens 2021; 10(10): 1330.
[http://dx.doi.org/10.3390/pathogens10101330] [PMID: 34684279]

[17]   Lee JE, Saphire EO. Ebolavirus glycoprotein structure and mechanism of entry. Future Virol 2009; 4(6): 621-35.
[http://dx.doi.org/10.2217/fvl.09.56] [PMID: 20198110]

[18]   Zheng H, Yin C, Hoang T, He RL, Yang J, Yau SST. Ebolavirus classification based on natural vectors. DNA Cell Biol 2015; 34(6): 418-28.
[http://dx.doi.org/10.1089/dna.2014.2678] [PMID: 25803489]

[19]   Lefebvre A, Fiet C, Belpois-Duchamp C, Tiv M, Astruc K, Aho Glélé LS. Case fatality rates of Ebola virus diseases: A meta-analysis of World Health Organization data. Med Mal Infect 2014; 44(9): 412-6.
[http://dx.doi.org/10.1016/j.medmal.2014.08.005] [PMID: 25193630]

[20]   Cantoni D, Hamlet A, Michaelis M, Wass MN, Rossman JS. Risks posed by reston, the forgotten ebolavirus. MSphere 2016; 1(6): e00322-16.
[http://dx.doi.org/10.1128/mSphere.00322-16] [PMID: 28066813]

[21]   Leroy EM, Kumulungui B, Pourrut X, *et al.* Fruit bats as reservoirs of Ebola virus. Nature 2005; 438(7068): 575-6.
[http://dx.doi.org/10.1038/438575a] [PMID: 16319873]

[22]   Health, V.D.o. EBOLA(EBOLA VIRUS DISEASE). 18.03.2024]; Available from:

https://www.vdh.virginia.gov/epidemiology/epidemiology-fact-sheets/ebola-ebola-virus-disease/

[23] Velásquez GE, Aibana O, Ling EJ, Diakite I, Mooring EQ, Murray MB. Time from infection to disease and infectiousness for ebola virus disease, a systematic review. Clin Infect Dis 2015; 61(7): 1135-40.
[http://dx.doi.org/10.1093/cid/civ531] [PMID: 26129757]

[24] Medicine, N.L.O. Ebola Virus. 18.03.2024]; Available from: https://www.ncbi.nlm.nih.gov/books/NBK560579/#:~:text=The%20mortality%20rate%20ranges%20from,is%20a%20feared%20biowarfare%20agent

[25] McElroy AK, Akondy RS, Davis CW, *et al.* Human Ebola virus infection results in substantial immune activation. Proc Natl Acad Sci USA 2015; 112(15): 4719-24.
[http://dx.doi.org/10.1073/pnas.1502619112] [PMID: 25775592]

[26] Ansari AA. Clinical features and pathobiology of Ebolavirus infection. J Autoimmun 2014; 55: 1-9.
[http://dx.doi.org/10.1016/j.jaut.2014.09.001] [PMID: 25260583]

[27] Jacob ST, Crozier I, Fischer WA II, *et al.* Ebola virus disease. Nat Rev Dis Primers 2020; 6(1): 13.
[http://dx.doi.org/10.1038/s41572-020-0147-3] [PMID: 32080199]

[28] Baseler L, Chertow DS, Johnson KM, Feldmann H, Morens DM. The pathogenesis of ebola virus disease. Annu Rev Pathol 2017; 12(1): 387-418.
[http://dx.doi.org/10.1146/annurev-pathol-052016-100506] [PMID: 27959626]

[29] Furuyama W, Marzi A. Ebola virus: pathogenesis and countermeasure development. Annu Rev Virol 2019; 6(1): 435-58.
[http://dx.doi.org/10.1146/annurev-virology-092818-015708] [PMID: 31567063]

[30] Coller BAG, Lapps W Jr, Yunus M, *et al.* Lessons learned from the development and roll-out of the rVSVΔG-ZEBOV-GP *Zaire ebolavirus* vaccine to inform marburg virus and *sudan ebolavirus* vaccines. Vaccines (Basel) 2022; 10(9): 1446.
[http://dx.doi.org/10.3390/vaccines10091446] [PMID: 36146524]

[31] America, I.D.S.o. Ebola Facts. 19.03.2024]; Available from: https://www.idsociety.org/public-health/ebola/ebola-resources/ebola-facts/

[32] Prevention, C.F.D.C.a. Ebola Disease. 19.03.2024]; Available from: https://www.cdc.gov/vhf/ebola/history/chronology.html

[33] Kourtis AP, Appelgren K, Chevalier MS, McElroy A. Ebola Virus Disease. Pediatr Infect Dis J 2015; 34(8): 893-7.
[http://dx.doi.org/10.1097/INF.0000000000000707] [PMID: 25831417]

[34] Church DL. Major factors affecting the emergence and re-emergence of infectious diseases. Clin Lab Med 2004; 24(3): 559-586, v.
[http://dx.doi.org/10.1016/j.cll.2004.05.008] [PMID: 15325056]

[35] Burrell CJ, Howard CR, Murphy FA. Epidemiology of viral infections.Fenner and White's Medical Virology. 5th ed. London: Academic Press 2017; pp. 185-203.
[http://dx.doi.org/10.1016/B978-0-12-375156-0.00013-8]

[36] Rugarabamu S, Mboera L, Rweyemamu M, *et al.* Forty-two years of responding to Ebola virus outbreaks in Sub-Saharan Africa: a review. BMJ Glob Health 2020; 5(3): e001955.
[http://dx.doi.org/10.1136/bmjgh-2019-001955] [PMID: 32201623]

[37] Yamaoka S, Ebihara H. Pathogenicity and virulence of ebolaviruses with species- and variant-specificity. Virulence 2021; 12(1): 885-901.
[http://dx.doi.org/10.1080/21505594.2021.1898169] [PMID: 33734027]

[38] LaBrunda M, Amin N. The emerging threat of ebola.Global Health Security: Recognizing Vulnerabilities, Creating Opportunities. Cham: Springer International Publishing 2020; pp. 103-39.
[http://dx.doi.org/10.1007/978-3-030-23491-1_6]

[39] Broadhurst MJ, Brooks TJG, Pollock NR. Diagnosis of ebola virus disease: past, present, and future. Clin Microbiol Rev 2016; 29(4): 773-93.
[http://dx.doi.org/10.1128/CMR.00003-16] [PMID: 27413095]

[40] Van Bortel T, Basnayake A, Wurie F, *et al.* Psychosocial effects of an Ebola outbreak at individual, community and international levels. Bull World Health Organ 2016; 94(3): 210-4.
[http://dx.doi.org/10.2471/BLT.15.158543] [PMID: 26966332]

[41] Henao-Restrepo AM, Camacho A, Longini IM, *et al.* Efficacy and effectiveness of an rVSV-vectored vaccine in preventing Ebola virus disease: final results from the Guinea ring vaccination, open-label, cluster-randomised trial (Ebola Ça Suffit!). Lancet 2017; 389(10068): 505-18.
[http://dx.doi.org/10.1016/S0140-6736(16)32621-6] [PMID: 28017403]

[42] Organization, W.H. Introduction to Ebola disease. 21.03.2024]; Available from: https://cdn.who.int/media/docs/default-source/ebola/introduction-to-ebola-disease.pdf? sfvrsn=26c6c127_1

[43] World Health Organization. Managing epidemics: Key facts about major deadly diseases. 2018 [cited 2024 24th Sep.]; Available from: https://www.who.int/publications/i/item/managing-epidemics-k-y-facts-about-major-deadly-diseases#:~:text=Overview.%20Epidemics%20of%20infectious

[44] CDC's response to the 2014–2016 Ebola epidemic—West Africa and United States. Morbidity and Mortality Weekly Report 2016; 65(3): 4-11. [MMWR].
[http://dx.doi.org/10.15585/mmwr.mm6503a4]

[45] Jones BA, Grace D, Kock R, *et al.* Zoonosis emergence linked to agricultural intensification and environmental change. Proc Natl Acad Sci USA 2013; 110(21): 8399-404.
[http://dx.doi.org/10.1073/pnas.1208059110] [PMID: 23671097]

[46] Bouchot A, Bordier M. The OIE strategy to address threats at the interface between humans, animals and ecosystems. Socio-Ecological Dimensions of Infectious Diseases in Southeast Asia 2015; pp. 275-91.
[http://dx.doi.org/10.1007/978-981-287-527-3_16]

[47] Pandey RU, Muralee SNS, Sah J. Bio-Diversity, ecosystem-health and their relation with pandemic. Integrated Risk of Pandemic: Covid-19 Impacts, Resilience and Recommendations, 2020: p. 61-86.
[http://dx.doi.org/10.1007/978-981-15-7679-9_3]

[48] Zinsstag J. One Health: the theory and practice of integrated health approaches. CABI 2021.
[http://dx.doi.org/10.1079/9781789242577.0000]

[49] Gebreyes WA, Dupouy-Camet J, Newport MJ, *et al.* The global one health paradigm: challenges and opportunities for tackling infectious diseases at the human, animal, and environment interface in low-resource settings. PLoS Negl Trop Dis 2014; 8(11): e3257.
[http://dx.doi.org/10.1371/journal.pntd.0003257] [PMID: 25393303]

CHAPTER 9

Lassa Fever Outbreak in Africa

**Navneet Arora[1], Rakesh Chawla[2], Abhishek Vijukumar[1], Amandeep Singh[3]
and Ranjeet Kumar[1,*]**

[1] *Department of Pharmacy Practice, I.S.F College of Pharmacy, Moga, Punjab-142001, India*

[2] *Department of Pharma Chemistry, University Institute of Pharmacy, Baba Farid University of Health Sciences, Faridkot, Punjab-151203, India*

[3] *Department of Pharmaceutics, ISF College of Pharmacy, Moga, Punjab-142001, India*

Abstract: Lassa fever, a viral hemorrhagic disease prevalent in West Africa, particularly in countries like Sierra Leone and Nigeria, is primarily caused by the Lassa virus (LASV). The multimammate rat (Mastomys natalensis) serves as the primary rodent reservoir for the virus. Human infection typically results from contact with the rodent's feces or through human-to-human transmission.

Although significant advancements have been made in understanding the virus's genetic structure, clinical presentation, and transmission, there remain critical unanswered questions regarding its pathophysiology, immunology, ecology, and epidemiology. Lassa fever outbreaks are common, and in densely populated areas, there is a risk of the virus evolving into new strains, while rodent reservoirs may continue to expand.

Due to the virus's potential for international spread and concerns surrounding bioterrorism, research efforts have intensified to develop medical countermeasures. While studies on possible treatments and vaccine candidates are ongoing, no approved vaccines or medications are currently available for human use. This review offers a comprehensive analysis of LASV virology, the progression of Lassa fever in patients, and current efforts to identify effective treatments.

Keywords: Epidemiology, Diagnosis, Lassa fever, LASV, Rodents, Ribavirin, Viruses.

INTRODUCTION

Lassa fever is a severe viral hemorrhagic illness endemic to West Africa, caused by the Lassa virus (LASV), a member of the **Adenoviridae** family. The clinical

---
* **Corresponding author Ranjeet Kumar:** Department of Pharmacy Practice, I.S.F College of Pharmacy, Moga, Punjab-142001, India; E-mail: ranjeetkumar2784@gmail.com

presentation of this zoonotic disease varies widely, ranging from mild or asymptomatic cases to severe multisystem involvement with high fatality rates. The primary source of LASV infection in humans is the multimammate rat (Mastomys natalensis), which sheds the virus in its urine and feces [1], as illustrated in Fig. (**1**).

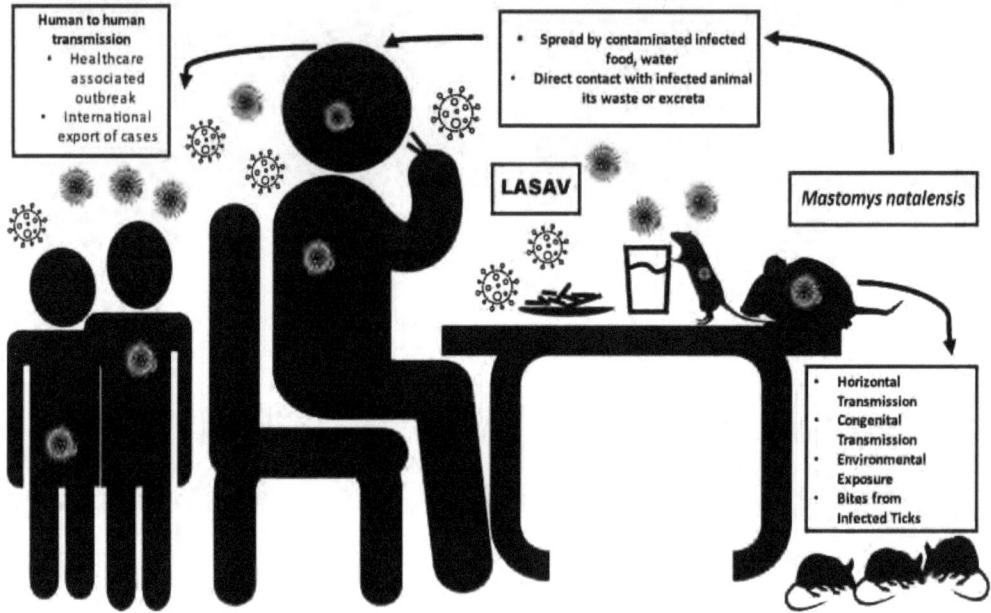

Fig. (1). "Transmission Pathways of Lassa Virus: From *Mastomys natalensis* Reservoir to Spillover and Human-to-Human Transmission".

Rodents, especially **Mastomys natalensis**, are the primary reservoir of the Lassa virus (LASV). LASV can spread among rodents via congenital or horizontal pathways. The virus can also infect other animal species, and ticks feeding on these animals are potential carriers. Exposure to these rodents or intermediate hosts, through their excretions or handling of infected animals, may cause LASV spillover. Human-to-human transmission can occur both at home and in medical facilities.

Epidemiologically, Lassa fever is prevalent in countries such as Sierra Leone, Nigeria, Liberia, and Guinea, where environmental conditions favor the proliferation of the rodent reservoir. Human infections occur through direct or indirect contact with rodent excreta, creating a complex chain of transmission. Person-to-person transmission, especially within healthcare settings, has contributed to amplifying outbreaks, highlighting the importance of nosocomial precautions in preventing the spread of the disease.

The clinical spectrum of Lassa fever ranges from mild to severe manifestations. Early stages resemble influenza-like symptoms, such as fever, headache, and general malaise [2]. However, severe cases may lead to respiratory distress, encephalopathy, hemorrhagic signs, and multi-organ failure. Mortality rates vary between outbreaks and regions, often reflecting the quality of healthcare infrastructure and access to medical interventions. Lassa fever poses a significant public health risk, with case mortality rates for hospitalized patients reported to approach 50%. Currently, there are no specific antiviral medications available for Lassa fever. Supportive care remains the cornerstone of treatment, addressing complications such as shock, organ failure, and fluid imbalances [3]. Early treatment with the broad-spectrum antiviral ribavirin has been shown to reduce mortality rates, although its effectiveness is limited by the challenges of early diagnosis and varying patient responses to treatment.

Efforts to develop vaccines against Lassa fever have gained momentum. Various vaccination strategies, including protein subunits and viral vectors, have shown promise in preclinical and early clinical trials [4]. These vaccines aim to stimulate protective immune responses against LASV, preventing or reducing the severity of the disease. While no vaccine has yet been approved for widespread use, ongoing research and clinical trials offer hope for the future implementation of vaccination strategies.

Diagnostic approaches for Lassa fever include both laboratory-based and field-friendly methods. Reverse transcription polymerase chain reaction (RT-PCR) remains the gold standard for diagnosing LASV infection due to its sensitivity and specificity. Additionally, serological tests that detect LASV-specific antibodies aid in diagnosing previous infections and assessing population exposure. Given the limitations of laboratory infrastructure in endemic regions, point-of-care tests are being developed to facilitate rapid diagnosis and timely management.

Lassa fever represents a complex interplay between a zoonotic virus, a rodent reservoir, and human susceptibility [5]. Human activities and environmental factors shape the disease's epidemiology, leading to a range of clinical outcomes. Despite the challenges of high case fatality rates, the absence of approved antiviral therapies, and sporadic outbreaks, research efforts are advancing our understanding of the virus's biology, developing medical interventions, and improving diagnostic strategies. These collective efforts hold promise for better preparedness, mitigation, and control of Lassa fever in endemic regions and beyond.

History

Lassa fever's history is closely tied to its discovery in the late 1960s. In 1969, two missionary nurses in the Nigerian state of Borno fell ill in the town of Lassa, marking the first recorded cases of Lassa fever. The nurses exhibited symptoms typical of viral haemorrhagic fever, including fever, malaise, sore throat, and muscle aches, which progressed to more severe manifestations such as bleeding and shock. Unfortunately, both nurses succumbed to the illness. The mysterious outbreak attracted the attention of medical researchers, leading to subsequent investigations. In 1970, scientists identified a new virus from the **Adenoviridae** family as the primary cause of the illness. This virus was named the Lassa virus (LASV), after the town where the first known cases were documented.

Following the virus's discovery, its origins and transmission dynamics were gradually elucidated. It was found that the virus is primarily maintained within the population of multimammate rats (**Mastomys natalensis**), which are widespread across West Africa. Human infections occur when individuals come into contact with virus-laden urine or faeces from these rodents, or with contaminated food or objects. Person-to-person transmission, particularly within healthcare settings, further contributes to the spread of the disease [6].

The name "Lassa" is derived from the town where the disease was first identified, following the common practice in medicine of naming infectious diseases after geographic locations. This approach provides context for the disease's origin. While naming diseases after their location can offer historical and geographical reference, it is important to approach such naming practices with sensitivity to avoid the potential stigmatization of specific regions or communities [7].

Since its discovery, Lassa fever has remained a significant public health concern in West Africa, with periodic outbreaks and sporadic cases. The severe impact of the disease, with its potential for high mortality, has spurred ongoing research aimed at understanding its epidemiology, pathogenesis, and potential interventions, including vaccines and treatments.

The squares on the map indicate the first occurrences of Lassa fever, documented in the Nigerian town of Lassa. The affected individuals were later transported to Jos. The Lassa virus (LASV) is known to exist in seven distinct lineages (I–VII) in West Africa. Circles represent major research institutions, including Kenema Government Hospital (KGH), the National Public Health Institute of Liberia (NPHIL), the Irrua Specialist Teaching Hospital (ISTH) in Owo, and Abakaliki. Redeemers University, home to the African Center of Excellence for the Genetics of Infectious Diseases (ACEGID), is also depicted [7]. In Fig. (**2**) the map of western Africa further illustrates the distribution of the seven LASV lineages, labeled with Roman numerals I through VII [7].

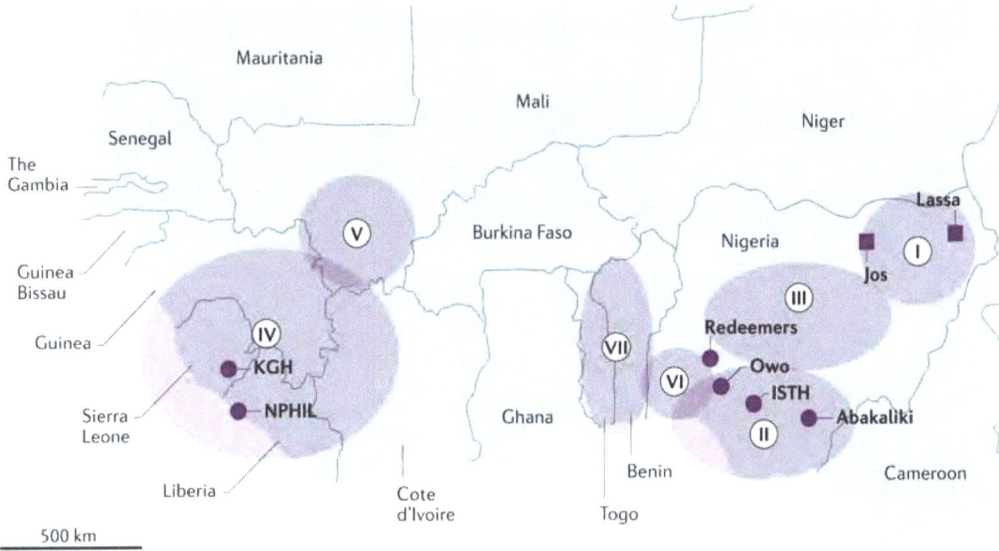

Fig. (2). Lassa fever prevalence and geography of outbreaks.

Lassa fever, caused by the Lassa virus, remains a persistent public health issue in West Africa, particularly affecting countries such as Ghana, Liberia, Guinea, Nigeria, and Sierra Leone. It is estimated that 300,000 to 500,000 cases occur annually, resulting in approximately 5,000 deaths. However, some estimates suggest that the number of cases may be as high as 3 million [7].

Epidemiology Challenges

Several factors complicate the accurate determination of Lassa fever's prevalence. These include the lack of essential diagnostic tools, inadequate public health surveillance infrastructure, and the concentration of cases around high-intensity sampling sites, all of which hinder precise incidence estimation.

Demographic Patterns and Geographical Distribution

Lassa fever shows a notable demographic bias, affecting females 1.2 times more frequently than males. Additionally, individuals in the 21-30 age group appear particularly vulnerable, indicating unique susceptibilities within this cohort. The disease is most prevalent in high-risk areas near West Africa's eastern and western borders, forming the so-called "Lassa belt," which includes Guinea, Nigeria,

Sierra Leone, and Liberia as of 2018. In Sierra Leone and Liberia, between 10-16% of hospitalized patients had Lassa fever by 2003, with case fatality rates ranging from 15% to 20%. Notably, the risk areas are not strictly delineated by biogeographical or environmental factors but are closely tied to the distribution of the multimammate rat, the primary carrier of the virus.

Regions such as Guinea (Kindia, Faranah, and Nzérékoré), Liberia (Lofa, Bong, and Nimba counties), Nigeria (around 10 out of the 36 states), and Sierra Leone (especially Kenema and Kailahun districts) are considered high-risk. In contrast, neighbouring countries like Ghana, Senegal, Mali, and the Central African Republic report a lower prevalence of Lassa fever [7]. Benin recorded its first cases in 2014, followed by Togo in 2016.

As of 2013, Lassa fever had rarely spread beyond West Africa, with only a few isolated cases confirmed in Europe. These imported cases carried a high fatality risk, primarily due to delayed diagnosis and treatment, stemming from a lack of familiarity with the symptoms [5-7].

COUNTRY-SPECIFIC OUTBREAKS

Nigeria

- **2018 Outbreak:** Eighteen states were affected by the worst Lassa fever epidemic in Nigerian history, resulting in 1,081 suspected cases and 90 confirmed deaths.
- **2019 Outbreak:** Nigeria recorded 810 cases and 167 deaths, corresponding to a case fatality rate of 23.3%.
- **2020 Outbreak:** By the ninth week of the pandemic, which began in January, there were 855 cases and 144 deaths, yielding a case fatality rate of 16.8%.
- **2021 Outbreak:** Two deaths were reported on December 8, 2021.
- **2022 Outbreak:** Between January 3 and January 30, 2022, 211 laboratory-confirmed cases, including 40 fatalities, were reported across 14 states and the Federal Capital Territory [7].

Liberia

- Liberia experiences periodic Lassa fever outbreaks, as the disease is endemic. Between January 2017 and January 2018, 91 suspected cases, 33 of which were laboratory-confirmed, were documented, with a case fatality rate of 45.4% [7].

Pathogenesis

The Lassa virus (LASV) closely interacts with the human immune system throughout the course of Lassa fever, resulting in various clinical manifestations.

LASV primarily infects immune cells like dendritic cells and macrophages, along with blood vessel endothelial cells, which leads to hallmark symptoms such as hemorrhaging and vascular leakage. The virus typically enters the human body through mucosal surfaces or skin breaks. After infecting immune cells, the virus spreads to other tissues and organs, such as the liver, spleen, and endothelial cells, by entering the bloodstream [8]. Fig. (**3**) provides Lassa fever distribution in Western Africa [36].

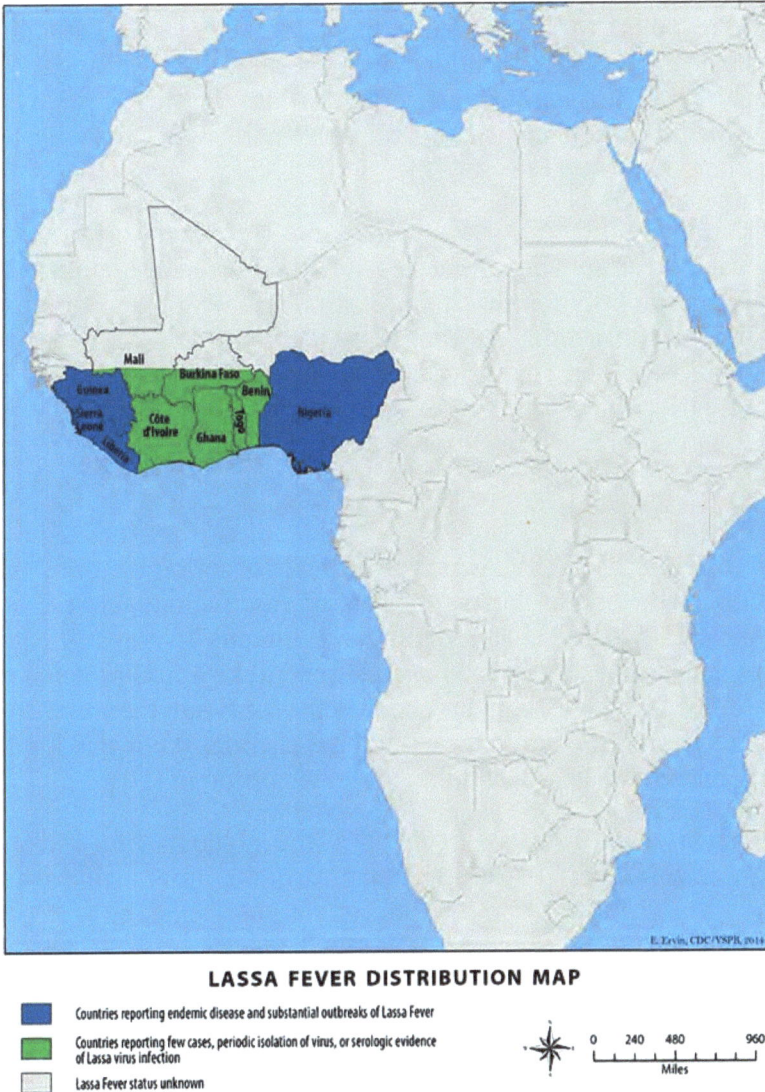

LASSA FEVER DISTRIBUTION MAP

Countries reporting endemic disease and substantial outbreaks of Lassa Fever

Countries reporting few cases, periodic isolation of virus, or serologic evidence of Lassa virus infection

Lassa Fever status unknown

Fig. (3). Lassa fever Distribution Map, the figure is taken from https://www.cdc.gov/vhf/lassa/index.html , the copyright belongs to Ervin, CDC, 2014.

One of the virus's significant characteristics is its ability to evade early immune responses, allowing it to establish infection undetected. Upon entering host cells, LASV replicates in the cytoplasm, releasing viral particles that infect neighboring cells and contribute to disease progression [8, 9]. The interaction between LASV and endothelial cells leads to increased vascular permeability, causing fluid leakage into surrounding tissues, which results in the hemorrhagic and edematous signs seen in severe cases.

The immune response to LASV can be both protective and damaging. While a strong immune response is essential for controlling the infection, an overactive response may lead to tissue damage, organ failure, and cytokine dysregulation, which can worsen systemic inflammation and contribute to the severity of the disease [8, 9].

Diagnosing LASV infection is challenging because early symptoms are nonspecific and overlap with other febrile illnesses. Laboratory methods like reverse transcription polymerase chain reaction (RT-PCR) and serological assays are necessary for confirming the diagnosis. While there is no specific antiviral treatment for Lassa fever, ribavirin has proven effective in reducing mortality if administered early. Supportive care, such as managing electrolyte imbalances, shock, and organ failure, is crucial for severe cases [8, 9].

Genetics of Lassa Virus

The genetic makeup of LASV, which is critical for its replication, transmission, and interaction with human hosts, consists of ribonucleic acid (RNA). LASV's genome comprises two single-stranded RNA segments known as the large (L) and small (S) segments. These segments encode several key viral proteins essential for the virus's lifecycle. The L segment encodes the viral polymerase, responsible for replicating the viral RNA, while the S segment encodes the matrix protein (Z), the glycoprotein precursor (GPC), and the viral nucleoprotein (NP).

One important aspect of LASV genetics is the glycoprotein precursor (GPC), which produces GP1 and GP2, proteins that form the virus's spikes. These spikes enhance the virus's ability to bind to and infect host cells and are recognized by the host's immune system, triggering antibody production [9, 10].

Genetic Variability

LASV exhibits genetic variability across different strains or lineages, which affects how the virus behaves, its virulence, and its interactions with the host immune system. These genetic differences may influence disease severity and the effectiveness of potential treatments or vaccines [10].

The genetic makeup of the human host also influences susceptibility to Lassa fever. Certain genetic variations may affect how an individual's immune system responds to the virus, impacting the likelihood of developing severe disease. Variants related to antiviral defense mechanisms, immune response regulation, and viral entry receptors can affect disease outcomes [10, 11].

Understanding the genetics of LASV is vital for developing diagnostics, vaccines, and treatments. Genetic research also aids in monitoring outbreaks and devising strategies for disease prevention and control.

Clinical Signs and Symptoms of Lassa Fever

Lassa fever presents a wide range of clinical signs and symptoms that can make diagnosis difficult, as they often overlap with other viral infections. Here's an overview of its manifestations and diagnostic techniques [12-15]:

- **Fever:** A high fever is one of the earliest and most prominent symptoms of Lassa fever. The fever may be gradual in onset and persist for several days.
- **General Malaise:** Patients often experience a sense of general discomfort, fatigue, and weakness.
- **Headache:** Intense headaches are a common symptom, often accompanying the fever.
- **Sore Throat:** Many patients report a sore or scratchy throat.
- **Muscle Aches:** Muscular pains and body aches, often referred to as myalgias, are common.
- **Cough:** A dry or productive cough may develop, accompanied by respiratory symptoms.
- **Nausea and Vomiting:** Gastrointestinal symptoms such as nausea and vomiting can occur.
- **Diarrhoea:** Some patients may experience diarrhoea.
- **Chest Pain:** Chest pain, especially during breathing, can be present.
- **Abdominal Pain:** Abdominal pain and discomfort may occur due to involvement of the gastrointestinal system.
- **Haemorrhagic Symptoms:** In more severe cases, haemorrhagic symptoms may appear, including bleeding from the gums, nose, or gastrointestinal tract.
- **Respiratory Distress:** Severe cases may lead to respiratory distress and difficulty in breathing.
- **Encephalopathy:** Some patients may experience confusion, neurological symptoms, and encephalopathy.

Not all individuals infected with the Lassa virus experience severe symptoms. In fact, many may have mild or even asymptomatic infections. However, in more severe cases, Lassa fever can escalate rapidly, leading to life-threatening complications such as multi-organ failure and shock. The disease becomes especially dangerous when hemorrhagic symptoms, such as bleeding from the gums or gastrointestinal tract, and organ failure occur.

Due to the non-specific and flu-like nature of early symptoms, diagnosing Lassa fever based on clinical signs alone is challenging. This is where laboratory studies become essential. Serological tests, like those for detecting specific antibodies, and molecular assays such as **reverse transcription polymerase chain reaction (RT-PCR)**, play a critical role in confirming the infection and differentiating it from other febrile illnesses. RT-PCR is particularly useful in identifying the viral RNA during the early, acute phase of the disease.

Early detection of Lassa fever is vital, not only to provide patients with the best chance for recovery through supportive care and treatments like **ribavirin**, but also to prevent the virus from spreading, especially among healthcare workers. Effective management of Lassa fever—through rapid diagnosis, timely medical intervention, and stringent infection control measures—greatly improves patient survival rates and reduces the overall impact of the disease on public health [12-15].

Diagnosis of Lassa Fever

Diagnosing Lassa fever involves a multifaceted approach due to its nonspecific initial symptoms. Clinicians rely on a combination of clinical evaluations, laboratory tests, and epidemiological data to confirm the diagnosis and assess disease severity. Here are the key diagnostic components [16-19]:

Clinical Evaluation

• Recognizing symptoms characteristic of Lassa fever within endemic areas is vital for suspicion.
• Patient history, including travel to endemic regions and potential exposure to rodents or infected individuals, is crucial.

Laboratory Testing

Various diagnostic tests help confirm Lassa fever infection and guide patient management:

Serological Tests

• **Enzyme-Linked Immunosorbent Assay (ELISA):** Detects antibodies (IgG for past exposure, IgM for current infection).
• **Immunofluorescence Assay (IFA):** Identifies LASV-specific antibodies using

fluorescent markers.

Molecular Tests

- **Reverse Transcription Polymerase Chain Reaction (RT-PCR):** Identifies viral RNA, allowing for rapid diagnosis during the acute phase.
- **Real-Time PCR:** Offers quantitative and real-time monitoring of viral RNA.
- **Virus Isolation:** Grows the Lassa virus from patient samples, though it requires specialized facilities and is technically demanding.
- **Antigen Detection Assays:** Rapid tests for viral antigens are in development to enhance point-of-care diagnosis.

Histopathology

- Less common, this method examines tissue samples for characteristic changes associated with LASV infection but poses biosafety challenges.

Importance of Rapid Diagnosis

Rapid diagnosis is essential for:

- Initiating appropriate treatment.
- Implementing infection control measures to prevent outbreaks.
- Distinguishing Lassa fever from other infectious diseases with similar symptoms (*e.g.*, other viral hemorrhagic fevers and malaria).

Due to the high biosafety requirements for handling LASV, diagnostic tests should be conducted in specialized laboratories, and healthcare workers must receive training to mitigate exposure risks [16-19].

CURRENT TREATMENTS, IMMUNOTHERAPEUTICS, AND VACCINES FOR LASSA FEVER

Clinical Treatment

Currently, there is no certified antiviral treatment specifically for Lassa fever. However, **ribavirin**, a broad-spectrum antiviral drug, has been shown to reduce mortality rates when administered early in the disease course [20, 21]. Here are the details:

- **Action:** Ribavirin inhibits viral RNA polymerase, which hampers viral replication. Its effectiveness is most pronounced with early administration.
- **Dosage:** The regimen typically includes an initial loading dose followed by a maintenance dose, although optimal dosing and duration are not fully established.

- **Efficacy:** Outcomes vary based on factors such as treatment timing and disease severity, with some severe cases showing limited response.

Safety and Side Effects

Ribavirin can have side effects, including:

- **Anemia:** Requires monitoring of blood counts during treatment.
- **Considerations for Specific Populations:** Extra caution is needed for certain groups, such as pregnant women [22-24].

Alternative and Combination Therapies

- **Favipiravir:** Shows greater efficacy than ribavirin in animal models and has been used in combination treatments [25, 26].
- **Arevirumab-3:** A monoclonal antibody cocktail that demonstrated effectiveness in preventing Lassa fever in non-human primates [27].
- **LHF-535:** A viral entry inhibitor with a favorable safety profile, focusing on blocking LASV entry via its envelope glycoprotein [28, 29].

Vaccine Development

Research into vaccines for Lassa fever has gained momentum, exploring various candidates [29]:

Types of Candidates

- **Viral Vectors:** Aim to stimulate protective immune responses against LASV.
- **Protein Subunits:** Designed to induce immunity and mitigate disease severity.

Promising Candidates

- **ML29 MOPV/LASV Live Reassortant:** A potential vaccine candidate currently under investigation [29].

Challenges

Vaccine development is complex due to LASV strain variability, the disease's immunological aspects, and the need for extensive safety and efficacy testing [30-32].

WHO Recommendations

The World Health Organization (WHO) has been leading the charge in the continuous battle against infectious diseases, partnering with other organizations to address unique health hazards like Lassa fever. The Lassa virus, which is the cause of Lassa fever, is a severe public health concern in West Africa, notably in Sierra Leone, Guinea, and Liberia [1-5, 12]. Once they understood how terrible the situation was, the Ministries of Health of these three countries, the World Health Organization, the United countries, the Office of the United States Foreign Disaster Assistance, and other dedicated partners founded the Mano River Union Lassa Fever Network [5-8].

At the heart of this collaborative effort lies the commitment to bolster the capacities of Guinea, Liberia, and Sierra Leone in combating Lassa fever. The primary focus revolves around the development and implementation of national prevention strategies tailored to the unique challenges posed by the virus. This multifaceted approach involves not only preventive measures but also advancements in laboratory diagnostics to facilitate swift and accurate identification of Lassa fever cases, thereby enabling a more targeted response.

Improving laboratory diagnosis is vital to the Mano River Union Lassa Fever Network [13-18]. The program recognizes the pivotal role of diagnostic tools in early detection and containment of the virus. As such, a comprehensive training initiative has been launched, encompassing areas such as laboratory diagnosis, clinical management, and environmental control. This training equips healthcare professionals with the necessary skills to efficiently identify and manage Lassa fever cases, laying the foundation for a more resilient and responsive healthcare system.

Moreover, the collaborative effort extends beyond immediate response measures. The program's purpose is to reinforce the three countries' total healthcare system, making them better ready to tackle not just Lassa fever but also other dangerous ailments. By investing in training and capacity-building, the initiative contributes to the development of a sustainable and adaptable healthcare system capable of addressing a spectrum of health threats.

The Mano River Union Lassa Fever Network exemplifies the importance of international cooperation in the face of global health challenges [12, 33-35]. By pooling resources, expertise, and knowledge, the participating entities are creating a synergistic response to Lassa fever, reflecting a commitment to collective health security. The WHO's involvement underscores its dedication to fostering partnerships that transcend borders, emphasizing the shared responsibility of the international community in safeguarding public health. As the collaboration progresses, the hope is not only to mitigate the impact of Lassa fever but also to fortify the region's resilience against future health threats [12, 35].

CONCLUSION

In summary, this review provides a comprehensive overview of the historical, pathological, and therapeutic landscape of Lassa Fever. While substantial progress has been achieved, the dynamic nature of viral diseases necessitates ongoing research to adapt to emerging challenges. To date, Favipiravir and ribavirin remain the primary antiviral treatment options for Lassa fever, although their effectiveness can be variable and dependent on various factors. Vaccine development efforts are ongoing, with promising candidates being evaluated in preclinical and early clinical stages. As the understanding of the Lassa virus and the immune response continues to evolve, advancements in treatment and vaccine strategies hold promise for improving outcomes and controlling the spread of Lassa fever. By fostering a deeper comprehension of Lassa Fever's complexities, we are better equipped to respond effectively, protect vulnerable populations, and ultimately pave the way for a future with reduced morbidity and mortality associated with this devastating infectious disease [35].

AUTHORS' CONTRIBUTION

Navneet Arora, and Abhishek Vijukumar are responsible for the drafting, editing and illustration of the book chapter. Dr. Ranjeet Singh is responsible for the correspondence with the editor.

REFERENCES

[1]   Happi AN, Happi CT, Schoepp RJ. Lassa fever diagnostics: past, present, and future. Curr Opin Virol 2019; 37: 132-8.
[http://dx.doi.org/10.1016/j.coviro.2019.08.002] [PMID: 31518896]

[2]   Richmond JK, Baglole DJ. Lassa fever: epidemiology, clinical features, and social consequences. BMJ 2003; 327(7426): 1271-5.
[http://dx.doi.org/10.1136/bmj.327.7426.1271] [PMID: 14644972]

[3]   Alli A, Ortiz JF, Fabara SP, Patel A, Halan T. Management of lassa fever: a current update. Cureus 2021; 13(5): e14797.
[http://dx.doi.org/10.7759/cureus.14797] [PMID: 34094756]

[4]   Hadi CM, Goba A, Khan SH, *et al.* Ribavirin for Lassa fever postexposure prophylaxis. Emerg Infect Dis 2010; 16(12): 2009-11.
[http://dx.doi.org/10.3201/eid1612.100994] [PMID: 21122249]

[5]   Raabe V, Koehler J. Laboratory diagnosis of lassa fever. J Clin Microbiol 2017; 55(6): 1629-37.
[http://dx.doi.org/10.1128/JCM.00170-17] [PMID: 28404674]

[6]   Watts G. Lily Lyman Pinneo. Lancet 2012; 380(9853): 1552.
[http://dx.doi.org/10.1016/S0140-6736(12)61871-6] [PMID: 23122238]

[7]   Monath TP. A short history of Lassa fever: the first 10–15 years after discovery. Curr Opin Virol 2019; 37: 77-83.
[http://dx.doi.org/10.1016/j.coviro.2019.06.005] [PMID: 31323506]

[8]   Yun NE, Walker DH. Pathogenesis of Lassa fever. Viruses 2012; 4(10): 2031-48.
[http://dx.doi.org/10.3390/v4102031] [PMID: 23202452]

[9]   Shieh WJ, Demby A, Jones T, *et al.* Pathology and pathogenesis of lassa fever: novel immunohistochemical findings in fatal cases and clinico-pathologic correlation. Clin Infect Dis 2022; 74(10): 1821-30.
[http://dx.doi.org/10.1093/cid/ciab719] [PMID: 34463715]

[10]   Southern PJ. Fields Virology. Philadelphia: Lippencott-Raven 1996; pp. 1505-19.

[11]   Bowen MD, Rollin PE, Ksiazek TG, *et al.* Genetic diversity among Lassa virus strains. J Virol 2000; 74(15): 6992-7004.
[http://dx.doi.org/10.1128/JVI.74.15.6992-7004.2000] [PMID: 10888638]

[12]   WHO. Lassa fever. World Health Organization, 2022. Available from: https://www.who.int/health-topics/lassa-fever#tab=tab_1

[13]   Knobloch J, McCormick JB, Webb PA, Dietrich M, Schumacher HH, Dennis E. Clinical observations in 42 patients with Lassa fever. Tropenmed Parasitol 1980; 31(4): 389-98.
[PMID: 7233535]

[14]   McCormick J B, Fisher-Hoch S P. Lassa fever. Arenaviruses I: the Epidemiology, Molecular and Cell Biology of Arenaviruses, 2002; 75-109.
[http://dx.doi.org/10.1007/978-3-642-56029-3_4]

[15]   Ilori EA, Furuse Y, Ipadeola OB, *et al.* Epidemiologic and clinical features of lassa fever outbreak in nigeria, january 1–May 6, 2018. Emerg Infect Dis 2019; 25(6): 1066-74.
[http://dx.doi.org/10.3201/eid2506.181035] [PMID: 31107222]

[16]   Panning M, Emmerich P, Ölschläger S, *et al.* Laboratory diagnosis of Lassa fever, liberia. Emerg Infect Dis 2010; 16(6): 1041-3.
[http://dx.doi.org/10.3201/eid1606.100040] [PMID: 20507774]

[17]   Demby AH, Chamberlain J, Brown DW, Clegg CS. Early diagnosis of Lassa fever by reverse transcription-PCR. J Clin Microbiol 1994; 32(12): 2898-903.
[http://dx.doi.org/10.1128/jcm.32.12.2898-2903.1994] [PMID: 7883875]

[18]   Bausch DG, Rollin PE, Demby AH, *et al.* Diagnosis and clinical virology of Lassa fever as evaluated by enzyme-linked immunosorbent assay, indirect fluorescent-antibody test, and virus isolation. J Clin Microbiol 2000; 38(7): 2670-7.
[http://dx.doi.org/10.1128/JCM.38.7.2670-2677.2000] [PMID: 10878062]

[19]   Hortion J, Perthame E, Lafoux B, *et al.* Fatal Lassa fever in cynomolgus monkeys is associated with systemic viral dissemination and inflammation. PLoS pathogens. 2024 Dec 9;20(12): e1012768.

[20]   Salam AP, Duvignaud A, Jaspard M, *et al.* Ribavirin for treating Lassa fever: A systematic review of pre-clinical studies and implications for human dosing. PLoS Negl Trop Dis 2022; 16(3): e0010289.
[http://dx.doi.org/10.1371/journal.pntd.0010289] [PMID: 35353804]

[21]   Carrillo-Bustamante P, Nguyen THT, Oestereich L, Günther S, Guedj J, Graw F. Determining Ribavirin's mechanism of action against Lassa virus infection. Sci Rep 2017; 7(1): 11693.
[http://dx.doi.org/10.1038/s41598-017-10198-0] [PMID: 28916737]

[22]   Furuta Y, Komeno T, Nakamura T. Favipiravir (T-705), a broad spectrum inhibitor of viral RNA polymerase. Proc Jpn Acad, Ser B, Phys Biol Sci 2017; 93(7): 449-63.
[http://dx.doi.org/10.2183/pjab.93.027] [PMID: 28769016]

[23]   Russmann S, Grattagliano I, Portincasa P, Palmieri V, Palasciano G. Ribavirin-induced anemia: mechanisms, risk factors and related targets for future research. Curr Med Chem 2006; 13(27): 3351-7.
[http://dx.doi.org/10.2174/092986706778773059] [PMID: 17168855]

[24]   Chiou HE, Liu CL, Buttrey MJ, *et al.* Adverse effects of ribavirin and outcome in severe acute respiratory syndrome: experience in two medical centers. Chest 2005; 128(1): 263-72.
[http://dx.doi.org/10.1378/chest.128.1.263] [PMID: 16002945]

[25]   Safronetz D, Rosenke K, Westover JB, *et al.* The broad-spectrum antiviral favipiravir protects guinea

pigs from lethal Lassa virus infection post-disease onset. Sci Rep 2015; 5(1): 14775.
[http://dx.doi.org/10.1038/srep14775] [PMID: 26456301]

[26]   Lingas G, Rosenke K, Safronetz D, Guedj J. Lassa viral dynamics in non-human primates treated with favipiravir or ribavirin. PLOS Comput Biol 2021; 17(1): e1008535.
[http://dx.doi.org/10.1371/journal.pcbi.1008535] [PMID: 33411731]

[27]   Raabe VN, Kann G, Ribner BS, *et al.* Favipiravir and ribavirin treatment of epidemiologically linked cases of Lassa fever. Clin Infect Dis 2017; 65(5): 855-9.
[http://dx.doi.org/10.1093/cid/cix406] [PMID: 29017278]

[28]   Mire CE, Cross RW, Geisbert JB, *et al.* Human-monoclonal-antibody therapy protects nonhuman primates against advanced Lassa fever. Nat Med 2017; 23(10): 1146-9.
[http://dx.doi.org/10.1038/nm.4396] [PMID: 28869611]

[29]   Larson RA, Dai D, Hosack VT, *et al.* Identification of a broad-spectrum arenavirus entry inhibitor. J Virol 2008; 82(21): 10768-75.
[http://dx.doi.org/10.1128/JVI.00941-08] [PMID: 18715909]

[30]   Salami K, Gouglas D, Schmaljohn C, Saville M, Tornieporth N. A review of Lassa fever vaccine candidates. Curr Opin Virol 2019; 37: 105-11.
[http://dx.doi.org/10.1016/j.coviro.2019.07.006] [PMID: 31472333]

[31]   Johnson DM, Cubitt B, Pfeffer TL, de la Torre JC, Lukashevich IS. Lassa virus vaccine candidate ML29 generates truncated viral RNAs which contribute to interfering activity and attenuation. Viruses 2021; 13(2): 214.
[http://dx.doi.org/10.3390/v13020214] [PMID: 33573250]

[32]   Müller H, Fehling SK, Dorna J, *et al.* Adjuvant formulated virus-like particles expressing native-like forms of the Lassa virus envelope surface glycoprotein are immunogenic and induce antibodies with broadly neutralizing activity. NPJ Vaccines 2020; 5(1): 71.
[http://dx.doi.org/10.1038/s41541-020-00219-x] [PMID: 32802410]

[33]   Branco LM, Grove JN, Geske FJ, *et al.* Lassa virus-like particles displaying all major immunological determinants as a vaccine candidate for Lassa hemorrhagic fever. Virol J 2010; 7(1): 279.
[http://dx.doi.org/10.1186/1743-422X-7-279] [PMID: 20961433]

[34]   Kainulainen MH, Spengler JR, Welch SR, *et al.* Protection from lethal Lassa disease can be achieved both before and after virus exposure by administration of single-cycle replicating Lassa virus replicon particles. J Infect Dis 2019; 220(8): 1281-9.
[http://dx.doi.org/10.1093/infdis/jiz284] [PMID: 31152662]

[35]   Garry RF. Lassa fever — the road ahead. Nat Rev Microbiol 2023; 21(2): 87-96.
[http://dx.doi.org/10.1038/s41579-022-00789-8] [PMID: 36097163]

[36]   https://www.cdc.gov/vhf/lassa/index.html , the copyright belongs to Ervin, CDC, 2014.

CHAPTER 10

Future Perspectives and Conclusion

Amandeep Singh[1,*], **Rakesh Chawla**[2] and **Tuhin James Paul**[3]

[1] *Department of Pharmaceutics, ISF College of Pharmacy, Moga, Punjab-142001, India*

[2] *Department of Pharma Chemistry, University Institute of Pharmacy, Baba Farid University of Health Sciences, Faridkot, Punjab-151203, India*

[3] *Department of Pharmacy Practice, ISF College of Pharmacy, Moga, Punjab-142001, India*

FUTURE PERSPECTIVES

The emergence of deadly viruses and their global outbreaks pose serious threats to public health and global economies. The COVID-19 pandemic, an unprecedented disaster in recent times, has impacted health, social structures, and economies worldwide. Both developed and developing nations grapple with its severe consequences [1, 2]. This marks the third coronavirus outbreak of the 21st century to cause a large-scale epidemic. In response, top priorities include developing new drugs, conducting clinical trials for existing medications, and designing effective vaccines [3, 4]. Additionally, identifying the natural animal reservoirs of these viruses and restricting the consumption of such animals is crucial. Lessons from past outbreaks, like SARS-CoV and MERS-CoV, highlight the importance of establishing animal models that mimic human disease for vaccine development. While the global approach focuses on isolating populations to stop the spread until a vaccine is created, challenges exist in rapid vaccine development and testing, emphasizing the need for international collaboration [5]. Proper hygiene practices can significantly reduce the incidence of COVID-19 and other hygiene-related diseases [6]. Studying past outbreaks, like the devastating Spanish Flu pandemic of 1918, continues to inform our approach to influenza today. Research on the reconstructed 1918 virus has provided invaluable insights into how pandemics emerge and escalate [7]. This knowledge also allows us to predict the potential dangers posed by novel pandemic viruses. A critical takeaway from past outbreaks is the continuous evolution of influenza viruses and their ability to develop resistance to antiviral medications. The rapid rise of oseltamivir resistance in seasonal H1N1 viruses serves as a stark reminder of this vulne-

* **Corresponding author Amandeep Singh:** Department of Pharmaceutics, ISF College of Pharmacy, Moga, Punjab-142001, India; E-mail: ad4singh@gmail.com

rability. Despite the clear medical need, the development of new influenza antivirals has been hampered by limited market potential due to the unpredictable nature of the influenza season. Additionally, the requirement for early treatment and limitations of diagnostic tests further complicates widespread use. Designing and conducting clinical trials for influenza antivirals also present difficulties due to the lack of accepted surrogate markers and the variable nature of symptoms. However, there are signs of renewed interest in influenza antiviral development due to unmet medical needs, rapid emergence of resistance, government funding, and the 2009 pandemic. Significant investments have been made in developing new antivirals, particularly for severely ill patients and those needing long-lasting treatment options. Additionally, a variety of novel drug candidates with unique mechanisms of action are under development. The successful development and approval of these drugs will broaden treatment options for all age groups and special populations. Combination therapy, as seen with HIV antivirals, holds promise for increased efficacy and reduced resistance development. Antiviral drugs targeting host factors offer further advantages by potentially reducing resistance and offering broad-spectrum activity against various respiratory infections [8]. Dengue fever, a mosquito-borne viral infection impacting millions globally, is another growing public health threat. Understanding the factors influencing its spread, such as climate change-induced alterations in weather patterns and mosquito breeding grounds, is crucial for developing effective prevention strategies [9]. Limitations of the currently available vaccine further complicate the fight against dengue. While promising new vaccine candidates are under development, long-term monitoring is necessary before widespread use [10]. Zika virus, a mosquito-borne flavivirus, has emerged as a significant public health concern due to its potential to cause severe congenital disabilities and autoimmune complications. Understanding the intricate interplay between the Zika virus and its host is essential for developing effective prevention and treatment strategies. Researchers are actively investigating several aspects of ZIKV-host interaction, including the mechanism of placental infection and viral persistence in immune-privileged sites. Additionally, researchers are exploring the role of non-coding RNAs during ZIKV infection and developing diagnostic tools, antiviral drugs, and vaccines. The fight against emerging viral threats requires a coordinated global response [11]. Researchers, pharmaceutical companies, policymakers, regulators, and funding agencies must work together to identify and implement effective global strategies. This includes controlling the spread of these viruses, mitigating associated complications, and ultimately eradicating these emerging threats. New human-derived models, such as organoids and organ chips, offer a significant advantage over traditional *in vitro* models for studying virus-host interactions. These advancements hold promise for providing deeper insights into viral mechanisms, ultimately aiding in the design of more targeted and effective therapeutics [12]. By simultaneously addressing knowledge gaps and developing a robust arsenal of tools, researchers can effectively combat these emerging public health threats [4]. The emergence of the 2009 H1N1 influenza pandemic underscored the critical importance of a "One Health" approach. This approach recognizes the interconnectedness of human, animal, and environmental health and is essential for effectively preventing and responding to future influenza pandemics. Several key lessons emerged from the 2009 pandemic. An effective global system for coordinated surveillance and response is necessary for the early detection and control of influenza outbreaks in animal populations. This minimizes threats to both human and animal health. Successful disease investigation and response require strong communication and collaboration between human and animal health professionals [13]. Increased surveillance for swine flu virus infections in occupational groups with close animal contacts, such as poultry and swine workers, is crucial for the early detection of new human cases. Protecting the health of these groups can significantly reduce human-t--human transmission. Standardizing the naming of influenza viruses and diseases is vital to avoid public confusion about risk factors and to prevent unnecessary economic impacts on food producers [14]. Fig. (1) provides the mortality rates (%) of the viral outbreaks with Ebola being the most lethal [2, 15-17].

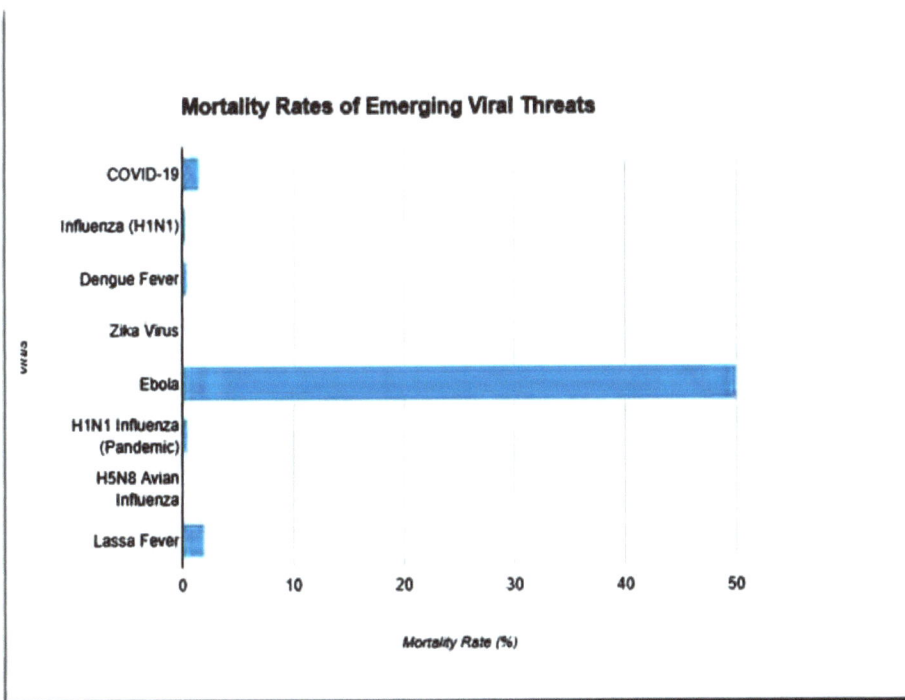

Fig. (1). Mortality rates of the viral outbreaks [2, 15-17].

Building trust with the food industry is essential to encourage early reporting of unusual animal diseases and participation in coordinated control efforts. Implementing biosecurity measures, sound management practices, and vaccination programs on swine farms can significantly reduce the spread of influenza viruses in animals. The timely development and availability of swine influenza vaccines targeting newly identified viral subtypes are crucial. Multidisciplinary research is needed to improve our understanding of influenza virus emergence, prevention, detection, and control in animals. This includes studying the links between animal production practices, infection risk, human-animal transmission, and food safety. Investments in training researchers and educators from diverse disciplines are essential for successful One Health initiatives. By implementing these lessons and fostering a collaborative One Health approach, we can be better prepared to prevent future influenza pandemics or respond to them more effectively. This will safeguard the health of both humans and animals on a global scale [16]. The HPAI(H598) virus underscores a dynamic situation with the geographic spread of the virus. Initially widespread in Africa and the Middle East, the viral outbreaks were reported from Nigeria and South Africa by November 2017, revealing that the virus demonstrated a capacity to infect both domestic poultry, including chickens and ducks, and wild bird species, such as ostriches, falcons, sparrows, crows, and doves. Notably, Taiwan reported no confirmed outbreaks in wild birds during this period. A significant finding concerns the presence of multiple subtypes of HPAI H5 viruses circulating in Asia. Outbreaks in Europe and Asia involved A (H5N8 explained the virus as containing genetic material from both HPAI and low pathogenic avian influenza (LPAI) viruses. This sheds light on the pathogenicity of the A(H5N8) strain. While exhibiting high mortality in chickens, the virus displayed lower virulence compared to A(H5N1) HPAI. Ducks and geese generally displayed mild illness or no symptoms. Studies suggest the possibility of transmission between certain wild bird species. Although no human cases were reported, the emergence of mutations in some Asian strains associated with increased binding to human-type receptors raises concerns about potential adaptation to humans. This underscores the importance of continued surveillance and monitoring of HPAI A(H5N8) to track its evolution and assess any potential increase in transmissibility or pathogenicity for humans [18]. Ebola vaccine research has made significant strides, with promising candidates reachingadvanced clinical trials. However, challenges persist in ensuring their efficacy, potency, durability, and affordability. Unlike earlier vaccines, current options necessitate a more comprehensive approach. This considers individual immune responses, local disease patterns, and the vaccines' effectiveness within specific communities. This knowledge can be a foundation for developing vaccines against emerging infectious diseases. Controlling future Ebola outbreaks requires a coordinated global response. Researchers, public health professionals, pharmaceutical companies, stakeholders, and funding agencies worldwide must collaborate on outbreak monitoring, ongoing research, and preparedness measures to effectively combat future threats [17]. Recent research on Lassa fever (LF), a severe viral hemorrhagic illness with high mortality rates in West Africa, highlights the urgent need for effective countermeasures. While antibody-based treatments show promise, their widespread availability is limited. Political instability in endemic regions further complicates control and management efforts. Vaccination represents the most viable long-term solution. Studies have demonstrated the potential of vaccines targeting the Lassa virus glycoprotein in animal models. However, significant challenges persist. Developing and producing a human vaccine necessitates overcoming political, scientific, and economic hurdles. Additionally, the high genetic diversity of the Lassa virus complicates efforts to create a broadly protective vaccine. Limited resources and the difficulty of conducting clinical trials in unstable regions further impede progress. Environmental factors also significantly influence Lassa fever transmission. Poor waste management, overcrowding, unsanitary living conditions, and seasonal changes are all believed to contribute to the spread of the virus. Improved sanitation practices, effective waste management strategies, and public health interventions targeting the zoonotic reservoir (rats) are crucial for mitigating these environmental risks [2]. A heatmap is explained for vaccine development in Fig. (**2**) [6, 8, 15] . A tabulated summarization of the book is also provided in Table **1**.

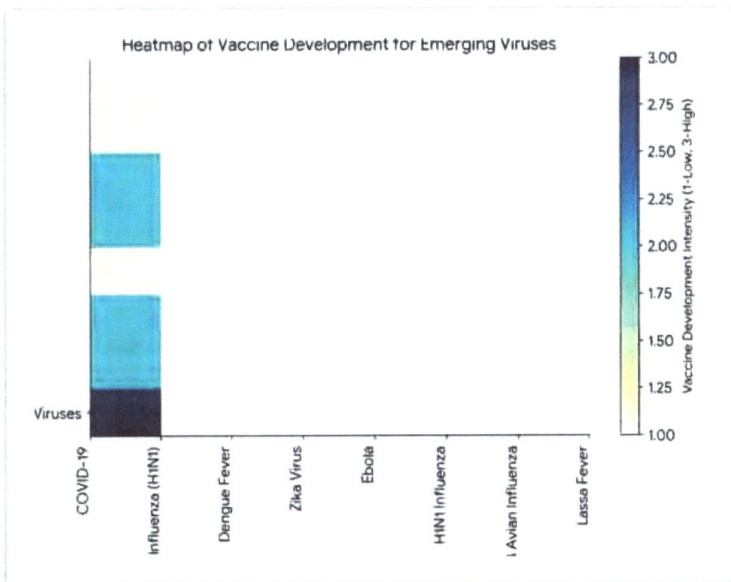

Fig. (2). Heatmap of vaccine development for emerging viruses [6, 8, 15].

Table 1. A tabulated summarization of the Book [1 - 3, 11, 16, 17].

Virus	Public Health Impact	Challenges	Strategies
COVID-19 (Coronavirus)	Devastating global pandemic impacting health, social structures, and economies.	Rapid vaccine development & testing, identifying animal reservoirs, international collaboration.	Hygiene practices, vaccine development, antiviral medication development.
SARS-CoV, MERS-CoV (Coronaviruses)	Past outbreaks highlight the importance of animal models for vaccine development.	Rapid Transmission of the virus, Identifying animal reservoirs, rapid mutation of the virus.	Establishing animal models for vaccine development.
Influenza	Highly contagious respiratory illness with seasonal outbreaks.	Rapid vaccine development & testing, resistance to antivirals.	Studying past outbreaks, vaccine development, research on new antivirals.
Dengue Fever	Mosquito-borne viral infection impacting millions globally.	Climate change impacting spread, limitations of current vaccine.	Understanding factors influencing spread, development of new vaccines.
Zika Virus	Mosquito-borne flavivirus, causing birth defects and autoimmune complications.	Understanding virus-host interaction for prevention & treatment.	Research on ZIKV-host interaction, diagnostics, antivirals, vaccines.
H1N1 Influenza Virus (Swine Flu)	Seasonal flu strain with Pandemic potential.	Unpredictable influenza seasons, early treatment requirement, lack of accepted surrogate markers for clinical trials.	Seasonal Flu anti-viral medication, anti-viral medication for therapy and management. Monitor for zoonotic transmission.
H598 Avian Influenza Virus	Highly pathogenic avian influenza, causing severe illness and death in birds.	Potential for zoonotic transmission and emergence of new pandemic strains.	Surveillance of HPAI viruses in poultry and wild birds, biosecurity measures on poultry farms, public health monitoring for zoonotic transmission
Ebola Virus	Severe hemorrhagic fever with high mortality rates	Individual immune responses are different, local disease patterns, and vaccine effectiveness within communities	Develop and ensure efficacy, potency, durability, and affordability of vaccines.
Lassa Fever	Severe viral hemorrhagic illness with high mortality rates in West Africa	Political instability in endemic regions, High genetic diversity of the Lassa virus, Limited resources and difficulty in conducting clinical trials.	Develop effective vaccines

CONCLUSION

The emergence and global spread of novel, highly pathogenic viruses pose a significant threat to global public health and economic stability. The COVID-19 pandemic serves as a stark reminder of the urgency for a coordinated global response to combat emerging infectious diseases. Key priorities include the development of efficacious vaccines and antiviral medications alongside efforts to identify and restrict the consumption of animal reservoirs harbouring these viruses. Invaluable insights into pandemic emergence and escalation have been gleaned from past outbreaks, such as the Spanish Flu and SARS-CoV. However, significant challenges persist in expediting vaccine development and testing, as well as designing and conducting robust clinical trials for novel antiviral drugs. Overcoming these hurdles necessitates international collaboration among researchers, pharmaceutical companies, policymakers, and funding agencies. The development of innovative human-derived models, like organoids and organ chips, holds promise for a deeper understanding of virus-host interactions, ultimately facilitating the design of more targeted therapeutics. The recent outbreaks of Dengue, Zika, Ebola, and Lassa fever further emphasize the critical need for a comprehensive global approach to controlling these emerging infectious diseases. This strategy should encompass continuous disease surveillance, implementation of effective preventative measures, and ensuring equitable access to affordable vaccines and treatments, even in regions facing political instability. By collaboratively addressing knowledge gaps, developing a robust arsenal of tools, and coordinating global response efforts, the international community can effectively combat these emerging public health threats and safeguard the well-being of populations worldwide. The book aims to highlight the lessons learned from recent epidemics, with a broad focus on various viral outbreaks. However, a complete picture of the pandemic's health, social, and economic impacts will only emerge after it subsides, informing our response to future outbreaks.

REFERENCES

[1]   Di Gennaro F, Pizzol D, Marotta C, *et al.* Coronavirus diseases (COVID-19) current status and future perspectives: a narrative review. Int J Environ Res Public Health 2020; 17(8): 2690.
       [http://dx.doi.org/10.3390/ijerph17082690] [PMID: 32295188]

[2]   Aloke C, Obasi NA, Aja PM, *et al.* Combating lassa fever in west african sub-region: progress, challenges, and future perspectives. Viruses 2023; 15(1): 146.
       [http://dx.doi.org/10.3390/v15010146] [PMID: 36680186]

[3]   Ji T, Liu Z, Wang G, *et al.* Detection of COVID-19: A review of the current literature and future perspectives. Biosens Bioelectron 2020; 166: 112455.
       [http://dx.doi.org/10.1016/j.bios.2020.112455] [PMID: 32739797]

[4]   Munjal A, Khandia R, Dhama K, *et al.* Advances in developing therapies to combat Zika virus: current knowledge and future perspectives. Front Microbiol 2017; 8: 1469.

[http://dx.doi.org/10.3389/fmicb.2017.01469] [PMID: 28824594]

[5]   Singh A, John OO, Bisola BB. Hand, foot, and mouth disease outbreak what you need to know. Infectious disorders-drug targets (formerly current drug targets-infectious disorders). 2023; 23(7): 77-81.

[6]   Sarkar C, Mondal M, Torequl Islam M, *et al.* Potential therapeutic options for COVID-19: current status, challenges, and future perspectives. Front Pharmacol 2020; 11: 572870.
[http://dx.doi.org/10.3389/fphar.2020.572870] [PMID: 33041814]

[7]   Nickol ME, Kindrachuk J. A year of terror and a century of reflection: perspectives on the great influenza pandemic of 1918–1919. BMC Infect Dis 2019; 19(1): 117.
[http://dx.doi.org/10.1186/s12879-019-3750-8] [PMID: 30727970]

[8]   Wathen MW, Barro M, Bright RA. Antivirals in seasonal and pandemic influenza--future perspectives. Influenza Other Respir Viruses. 2013;7 Suppl 1(Suppl 1): 76-80.

[9]   Idris F, Ting DHR, Alonso S. An update on dengue vaccine development, challenges, and future perspectives. Expert Opin Drug Discov 2021; 16(1): 47-58.
[http://dx.doi.org/10.1080/17460441.2020.1811675] [PMID: 32838577]

[10]   Soneja S, Tsarouchi G, Lumbroso D, Tung DK. A review of dengue's historical and future health risk from a changing climate. Curr Environ Health Rep 2021; 8(3): 245-65.
[http://dx.doi.org/10.1007/s40572-021-00322-8] [PMID: 34269994]

[11]   Lee JK, Shin OS. Advances in Zika virus–host cell interaction: Current knowledge and future perspectives. Int J Mol Sci 2019; 20(5): 1101.
[http://dx.doi.org/10.3390/ijms20051101] [PMID: 30836648]

[12]   Omosigho PO, John OO, Adigun OA, Hassan HK, Olabode ON, Micheal AS. The re-emergence of diphtheria amidst multiple outbreaks in nigeria. infectious disorders-drug targets (formerly current drug targets-infectious disorders). 2024; 24(4): 20-8.
[http://dx.doi.org/10.2174/0118715265251299231117045940]

[13]   Pappaioanou M, Gramer M. Lessons from pandemic H1N1 2009 to improve prevention, detection, and response to influenza pandemics from a One Health perspective. ILAR J 2010; 51(3): 268-80.
[http://dx.doi.org/10.1093/ilar.51.3.268] [PMID: 21131728]

[14]   Berridge V, Taylor S. The problems of commissioned oral history: the swine flu'crisis' of 2009. Oral Hist (Colch) 2019; 86-94.

[15]   Carrillo-Hernández MY, Ruiz-Saenz J, Martínez-Gutiérrez M. Coinfection of zika with dengue and chikungunya virus zika virus biology, Transmission, and Pathology. Elsevier 2021; pp. 117-27.
[http://dx.doi.org/10.1016/B978-0-12-820268-5.00011-0]

[16]   Mansoor S, Maqbool I. Swine flu a seasonal pandemic, symptoms, diagnostics and prevention. Rev Med Microbiol 2019; 30(4): 200-4.
[http://dx.doi.org/10.1097/MRM.0000000000000183]

[17]   Malik S, Kishore S, Nag S, *et al.* Ebola virus disease vaccines: development, current perspectives & challenges. Vaccines (Basel) 2023; 11(2): 268.
[http://dx.doi.org/10.3390/vaccines11020268] [PMID: 36851146]

[18]   Brown I, Kuiken T, Mulatti P, *et al.* Avian influenza overview September - November 2017. EFSA J 2017; 15(12): e05141.
[PMID: 32625395]

SUBJECT INDEX

A

Acute 4, 6, 8, 9, 29, 39, 45, 94, 97, 98
  hepatitis infection 6
  pancreatitis (AP) 8, 9
  respiratory distress syndrome (ARDS) 4,
    29, 39, 45, 94, 97, 98
Anti-inflammatory drugs 81
Antibiotic therapy 46
Antibodies 5, 7, 10, 11, 30, 42, 46, 70, 75, 81,
    94, 97, 110, 112, 143
  anti-influenza 46
  monoclonal 30, 46, 81
Antibody 60, 61
  -dependent enhancement 61
  tests, indirect immunofluorescent 60
Antigen detection assays 144
Antihistamines 80
Antiviral 8, 12, 29, 38, 45, 46, 48, 60, 80, 82,
    83, 90, 91, 95, 98, 101, 105, 112, 114,
    136, 141, 142, 150, 151, 155, 156
  activity 82
  agents 60, 80
  defense mechanisms 142
  drugs 12, 83, 90, 91, 98, 105, 151
  medication development 155
  medications 8, 38, 45, 46, 95, 101, 112,
    114, 136, 150, 156
  treatments 29, 48, 60, 141
Arboviruses 6, 7
Assay, enzyme-linked immunosorbent 60, 143
Autoimmune 78, 79
  disorder 79
  nerve disorder 78

B

Bacterial 11, 83, 97
  Artificial chromosomes 83
  infections 11, 97
Barré syndrome 71
Bleeding 5, 59, 122

gums 5, 59
problems 122
Blood 6, 7, 72
  meals 72
  transfusions 6, 7
Breathing 4, 14, 119
  difficulties 4, 119
  machines 14
Breathlessness 5
Broad-spectrum 144, 151
  activity 151
  antiviral drug 144
Bronchoscopy 4, 26

C

Cardiac resuscitation 26
Cell(s) 10, 30
  -intermediated immunity 10
  mesenchymal stem 30
Co-infections, bacterial 46, 47
Communities 12, 13, 31, 34, 119, 120, 123,
    124, 125, 127, 130, 137, 153, 155
  affected 119, 120, 124, 125
Conditions 3, 4, 5, 10, 28, 54, 98
  climate 4
  severe skin 98
Contaminated food 137
Coronavirus 23, 24, 25, 27, 33, 150, 155
  disease 24, 33
  outbreak 150
  pathogenic 24
Corticosteroid treatment 45
Coughs, dry 4
COVID-19 14, 24, 33, 34, 39, 108, 150, 156
  infection 24
  outbreak 39
  pandemic 14, 33, 34, 108, 150, 156
  respiratory illness 24
  virus 33
Cytokine(s) 29, 30, 44, 76, 141
  dysregulation 141

Amandeep Singh (Ed.)
All rights reserved-© 2025 Bentham Science Publishers

www.ingramcontent.com/pod-product-compliance
Lightning Source LLC
Chambersburg PA
CBHW041442210326
41599CB00004B/108